Quick-Start Guide

SURVIVING
AN URBAN
DISASTER

The Survival Essentials Made Easy
Small Steps, Big Results

RICHARD DUARTE

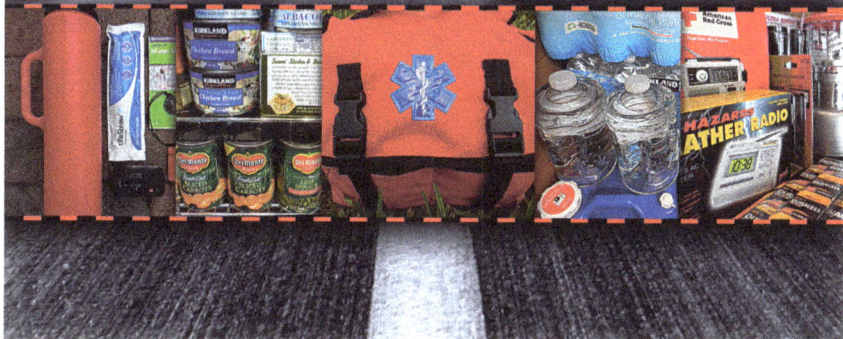

Surviving an Urban Disaster: Quick-Start Guide
Copyright © 2014 by Richard Duarte
Photographs © 2014 by Richard Duarte

ISBN-10: 1937660400
ISBN-13: 978-1-937660-40-6
Library of Congress Control Number: 2014951389

Publisher:

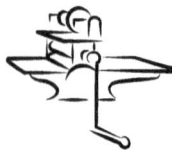

HERITAGE PRESS
PUBLICATIONS

Heritage Press Publications, LLC
PO Box 561
Collinsville, MS 39325

Editor: Hanne Moon
Cover/Interior Design: Lisa Thomson, BZ Studio

Contents

Author/Publisher's Note/Disclaimer

The information and other materials (collectively "Materials") contained in this book were obtained from sources believed to be reliable and accurate. The Materials may, however, contain inaccuracies or errors. The publisher and author make no representations about the accuracy, reliability, completeness, or timeliness of the Materials or about the results to be obtained from using the Materials. Neither the author, nor the publisher, shall be liable for any loss or damage allegedly arising from any information or suggestions contained in this book, and assume no liability for any incidents or injuries resulting from the use or misuse of the Material. Neither the author, nor the publisher, is engaged in providing professional advice or services to the individual reader. The Materials provided are for illustration and/or informational purposes only, and are not, nor are they intended to provide legal, medical, or any type of professional or lifesaving advice. The reader should consult with an appropriate professional regarding their individual situation. Any use of the information contained in this book shall be solely at the reader's risk. The possession, ownership, and use of firearms are governed by State and Federal laws. Readers should consult the applicable laws in their jurisdiction before buying, possessing, using, or otherwise engaging in any activities involving a firearm. If the reader has any doubts as to the applicable laws where they live, they should consult legal counsel. Comments and opinions expressed in this book represent the personal views of the individuals to whom they are attributed and are not necessarily those of the publisher or author, who make no guarantee or warranty, express or implied, regarding the reliability, accuracy, or completeness of the Materials. Any similarity or resemblance to any real persons, living or dead, actual facts, or places is purely coincidental, and not intentional.

Introduction

Every year countless natural and man-made disasters threaten our safety, potentially disrupting life as we know it. In the aftermath of any crisis, our access to food, water, medical attention, and vital public services can be quickly compromised. After just a few days without these life-sustaining resources, the world around us can become unrecognizable.

If tomorrow you woke up to a major disaster, would you know what to do? Would you have the necessary skills and supplies to survive? Would you even be able to keep yourself and your loved ones safe? Or, would you become just another name on a long list of victims?

Surviving an urban disaster requires advance planning, thoughtful preparations, and diverse skills. But, while many of us agree that "being prepared" saves lives, few of us actually do anything about it. (It's estimated that less than 1 percent of the U.S. population is prepared for a disaster or public emergency.) For some, it's a lack of time, money, and/or know-how. For others, life's concerns and hectic daily demands leave little room for much else. Regardless of the reasons (excuses), it all leads to the same conclusion—at any given moment 99 percent of the population is exposed, vulnerable, and unprepared to face the harsh realities. This unreasonable complacency should be unacceptable to most rational people.

Why This Guide?

The primary purpose of this guide is to help you get prepared quickly and easily. It summarizes the survival essentials in an abbreviated and user-friendly format—it's a quick-start guide for beginners and a handy reference for the more advanced. Getting prepared is actually pretty simple once you focus on the real-world survival basics and ignore the myths and extremes that are more entertainment than fact. The following pages are packed with practical information you need to know, without any sensationalism, fear mongering, or drama.

What to Expect

Each section of this guide is organized into easy-to-follow segments:

- ***What You Need to Know***—The survival basics presented in a clear, concise, user-friendly format.

- ***What You Need to Do***—Simple step-by-step guidelines to help you get started with minimum effort, time, and expense.

- ***What You Need to Get***—Comprehensive lists of supplies to buy and store.

- ***Quick Tips, Ideas and Information***—Fast and easy access to the facts you need.

- ***Pocket Reference/Survival at a Glance***—For fast access to important information, measurements, and details.

You don't need to be a survival "expert" to be prepared. You can get started in as little as a few hours; you just need to focus on the things that really matter.

What It's Not

This guide is not meant to be your only source of information. It's a starting point to get you thinking and moving in the right direction. Preparedness is a lifestyle, and not something you can do over a long weekend and then forget about. You need to work at it, and even though skills are always better than "stuff," none of it will matter much if you never get started. Lastly, this is not about *gloom and doom,* or end-of-world scenarios—it's about taking control and making reasonable, rational, common sense decisions based on knowledge and logic, not fear.

Using Your Guide—Getting Started

The information on these pages comes from real-life experience, extensive research, and trial and error—in other words, much of the heavy lifting has already been done for you. You don't need to read the entire guide to begin your preparations; you can work on it one section at a time in whatever order you like. But, no matter how you choose to proceed, the important thing is to get started.

Nothing any of us can do will ever prevent bad things from happening. The very best we can hope for is to have a fighting chance. When the moment arrives, you will either be prepared or you won't…the choice is yours. Being prepared will not only significantly increase your chances for survival, but will bring you peace of mind. Knowing this, what are you waiting for?

Stay Safe & Be Prepared
Richard Duarte

Quick Prep Tip

Nothing is ever 100 percent, but even some very basic preparations and planning will dramatically increase your chances for survival during a disaster.

Urban Survival Basics

Being "prepared" can mean different things to different people. This lack of clarity often creates confusion and complications. But, in reality, preparedness is quite simple. All disasters have one common underlying truth—in order to survive, you need the survival basics; these are the essential building blocks of any viable survival plan. I call these basics the **Core Survival Elements (CSE)**:

- Water

- Food

- First Aid and Medical

- Personal Security and Self-Defense

- Knowing When to Stay Put and When to Get Out

- Hygiene and Sanitation

No matter who you are or what urban catastrophe comes knocking at your door, you'll need the CSE to survive; these common-sense essentials increase your chances of surviving an urban disaster. If you're going to devote time, effort, and money to getting prepared, doesn't it make sense to start with (and stay focused on) the basics? By understanding and applying this simple truth, you'll take a huge step towards getting ready for just about any crisis.

Quick Prep Tip

One common mistake people make in any survival situation is to vastly underestimate the risks and to overestimate their abilities.

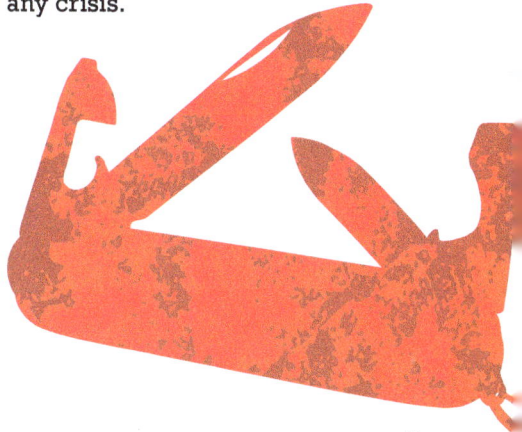

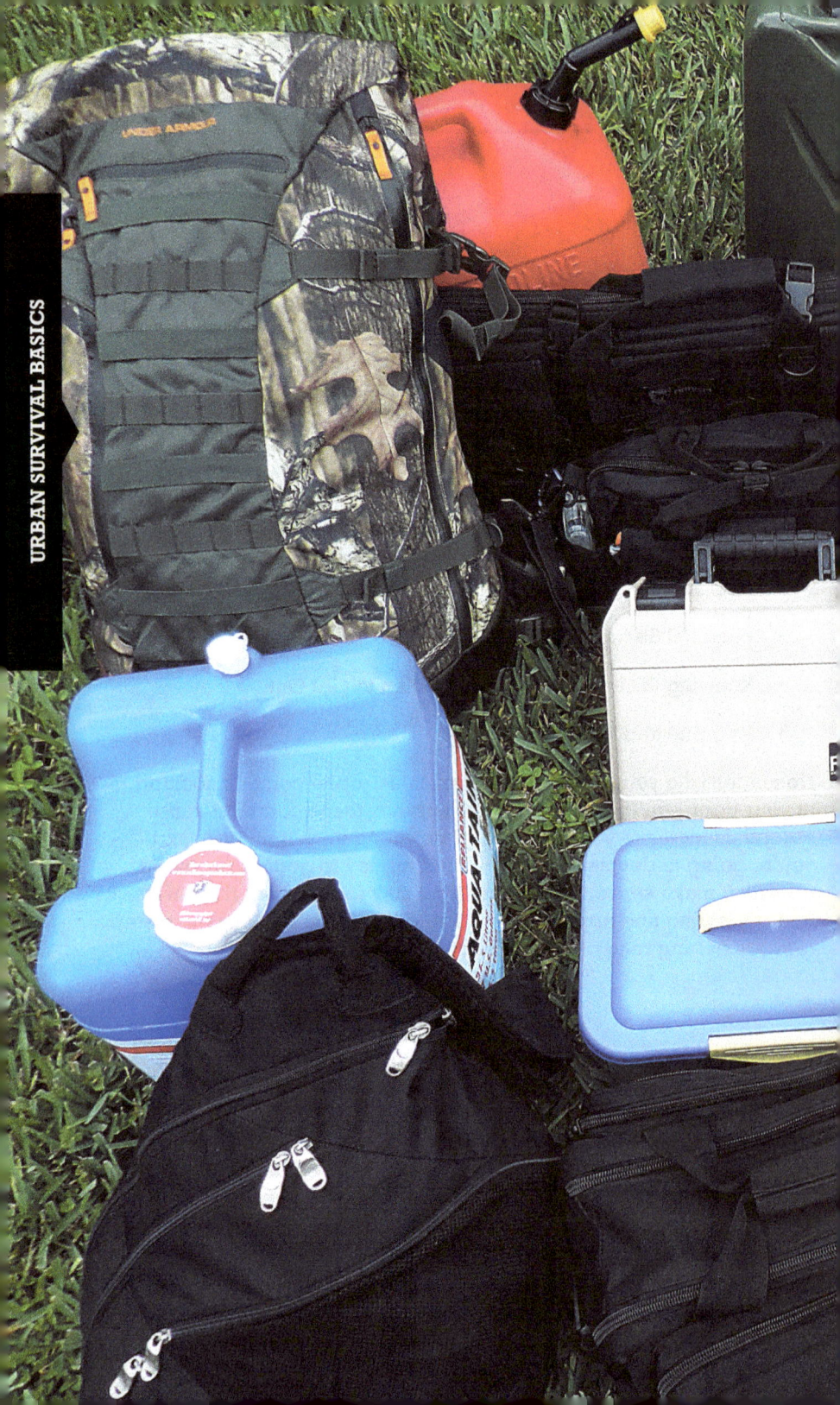

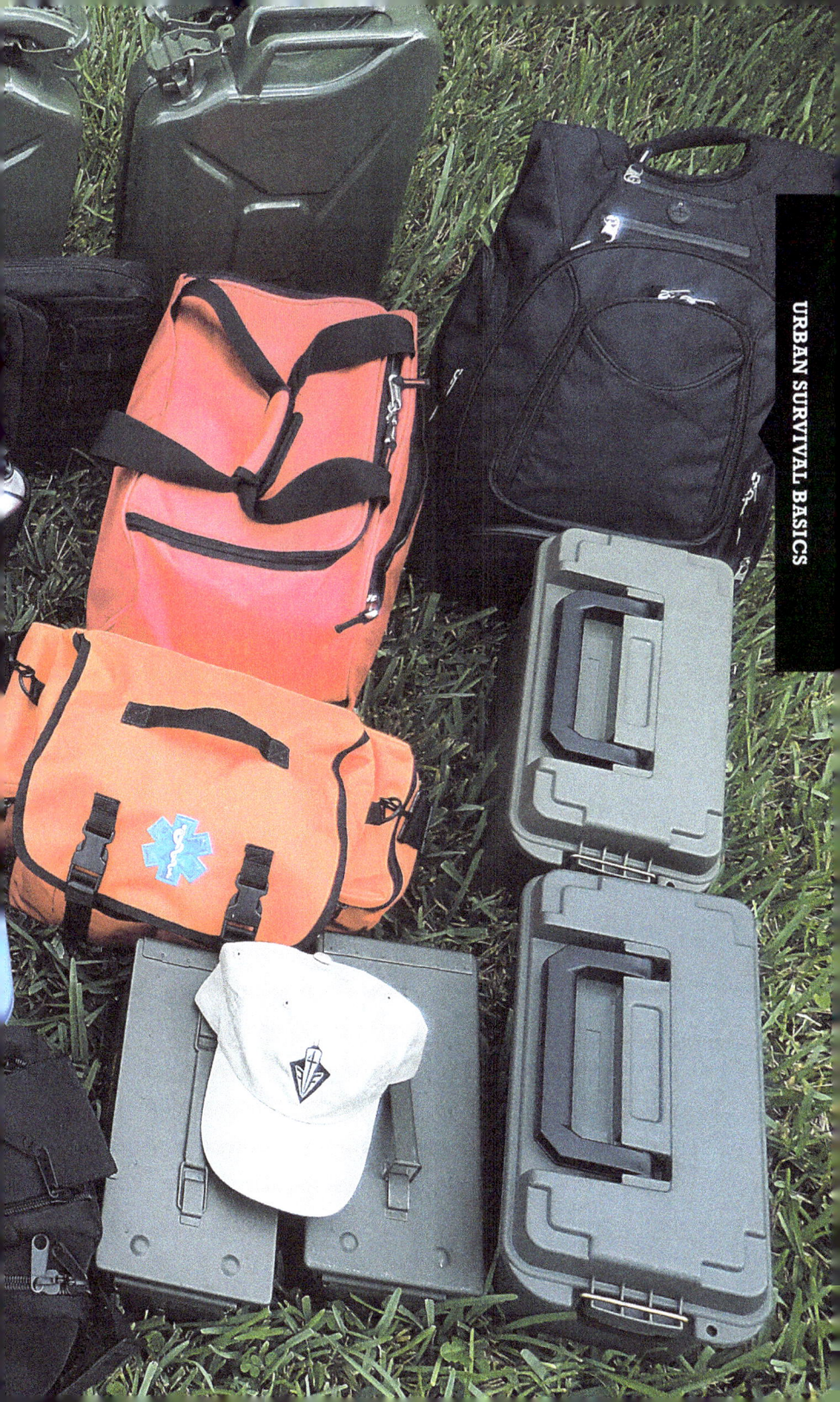

SURVIVAL AT A GLANCE

Urban Preparedness in 10 Simple Steps:

1. ***Expand Your Options*** – Being prepared and having a plan increases your range of available options when you need them most...before, during, and after a crisis.

2. ***Focus on the Core Survival Elements*** – Food, water, first aid, security/self-defense, sanitation/hygiene, and knowing when to stay put and when to get out. These are the things that will keep you alive.

3. ***Don't Focus on or Prepare for Specific Threats*** – Threats are unpredictable and outside your control. Being prepared is not about trying to predict the future. It's about expanding your options and making the most of your available resources.

4. ***Security and Self-Defense*** – No amount of food, water, or other resource will matter much if you're dead or seriously injured. Security and self-defense will always be a top priority.

5. ***Redundancy is King*** – If you just have one of anything, you have nothing. Always have a back-up for anything worth having. This includes supplies, equipment, and plans.

6. ***Separate Fact from Fiction*** – Your survival plans and preparations need to be realistic. Keep the fantasy where it belongs in video games, movies, and on TV.

7. ***Knowledge/Skills Trump "Stuff"*** – Storing supplies

without developing the corresponding knowhow is hoarding, not preparing. Knowledge and skills will always be better than "stuff."

8. ***The Mind is the Most Valuable Survival Resource*** – The ability to accurately assess a situation and make solid decisions is key and will dramatically improve your chances for survival. Prepare the mind!

9. ***Preparedness is a Lifestyle*** – Make it a part of your routine and incorporate it into your everyday life, but don't obsess. Balance and rational thinking are the keys to success.

10. ***Take Control, Turn Thought into Action*** – Think it through and plan, but also make sure to take action. Do the very best you can within your limitations and abilities, but get started. Always keep improving and refining your plans and preparations.

URBAN SURVIVAL BASICS

Quick Prep Tip

Never focus on specific threats. Instead, concentrate your efforts on securing the CSE. The survival basics will serve you well, no matter what disaster comes your way. Trying to anticipate and prepare for specific threats is impractical and will leave you exposed to all those things that you didn't (or couldn't) anticipate.

Quick Prep Tip

Some people mistakenly believe that different disasters require different preparations. By focusing on the survival basics, however, you are actually preparing for all events— known or unknown.

FOOD

WHAT TO KNOW

- Most people will not survive for more than three weeks without food. After just a few days without food, health, energy levels, and morale will all start to deteriorate significantly.

- A natural or man-made crisis can potentially disrupt the food supply chain; people in urban and suburban areas are especially vulnerable. Even a short-term disruption can be disastrous.

- Local food retailers typically maintain an inventory consisting of 72 hours or less on their shelves, but pre-disaster panic buying and hoarding can empty store shelves within hours of any major crisis.

- Hunger and panic will cause otherwise rational, law-abiding people to commit acts of desperation as they search for food anywhere they can find it. Having an adequate food supply will allow you to avoid the chaos outside your doors.

- Your first food priority is to ensure you can feed yourself and your loved ones during a crisis. It's all about getting enough calories.

Quick Prep Tip

Rice with beans is the ultimate survival food. Beans are loaded with antioxidants, fiber, and minerals. When combined with rice, beans provide an excellent high-quality protein source. Rice and beans are affordable and store well with minimal preparation.

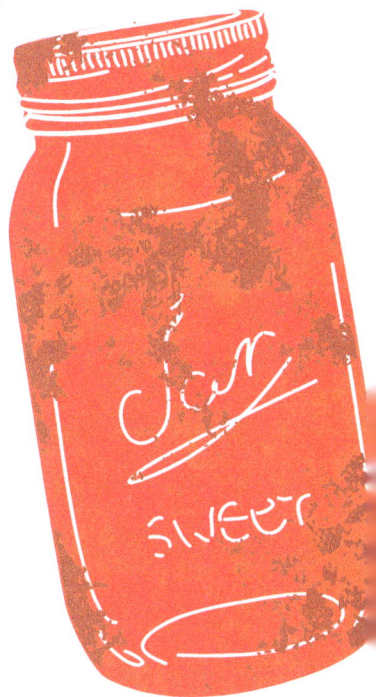

...ential Assortment

Made with real beef and chicken!

0g Trans Fat per Serving!

Assortment Contains:
4 Rice & Chicken
4 Chili Mac with Beef
4 Spaghetti with Meat Sauce

Just Add Water!

Ideal for emergency preparedness, camping, or backpacking

12 POUCHES/32 SERVINGS   NET WT 62.79 OZ (3.92 LB) 1.8Kg

Mountain House

Just In Case...

Classic Assortment

Made with real beef and chicken!

0g Trans Fat per Serving!

Assortment Contains:
2 Beef Stroganoff with Noodles
2 Lasagna with Meat Sauce
2 Chicken Teriyaki with Rice
2 Noodles and Chicken
2 Beef Stew
2 Granola with Blueberries

Just Add Water!

Ideal for emergency preparedness, camping, or backpacking

12 POUCHES/29 SERVINGS   NET WT 55.24 OZ (3.45 LB) 1.56Kg

smmmile...

15 packs
of the cheesiest

15-7.25 OZ (206g) BOXES, NET WT 6 LB 12.75 OZ (3.09kg)

TRADER GIOTTO'S
ITALIAN
BREADSTICKS

365
ORGAN...

Quin...

KIRKLAND
ALMONDS
US #1 SUPREME WHOLE

3 LBS.

NET WT 1.36KG (3 LB)

Barilla

ELBOWS
PERFECTION IN 7-8 MINUTES

#1 BRAND OF PASTA

2013

New!

13

MUELLER'S

— 100% —
Whole Grain

PENNE

ROMAN...

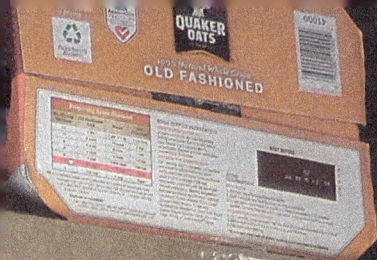
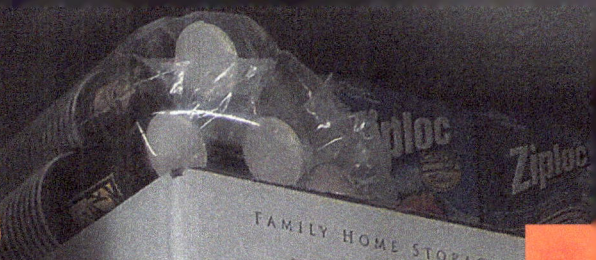
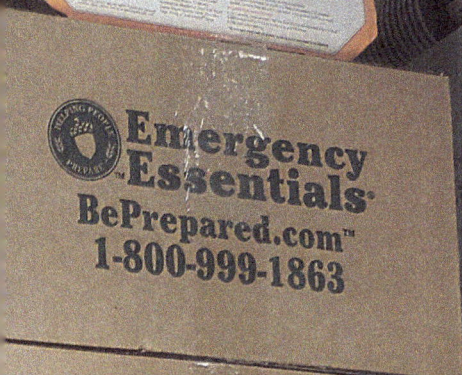
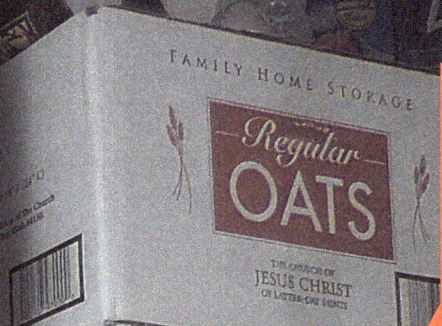
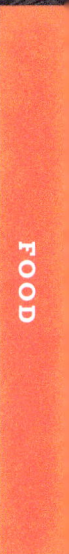
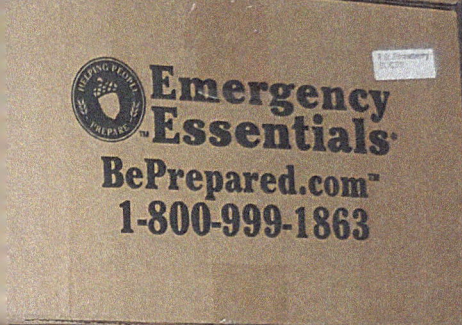
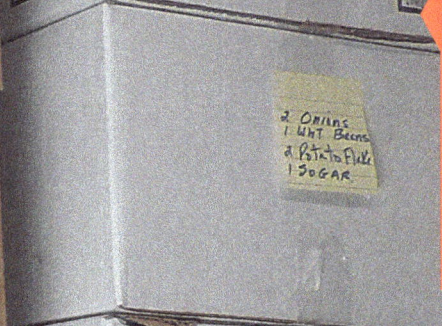
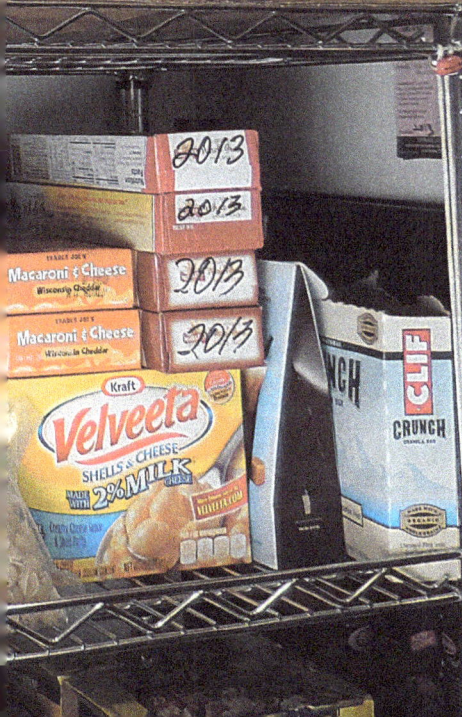
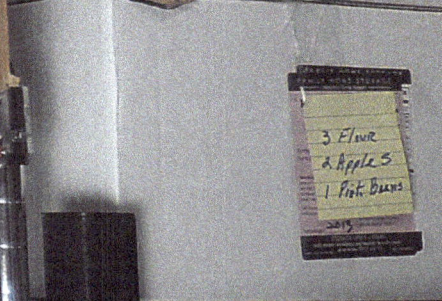
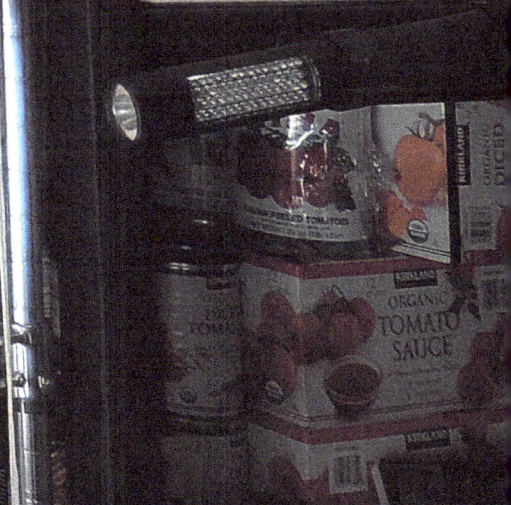

FOOD

- You need a viable food management plan to make the most of your food stores.

- Food labeling dates can be confusing and are often misinterpreted. Knowing what these dates actually mean and using them correctly can save you time and money.

- Digestion of protein-rich foods requires extra water. Store sufficient water for your needs.

WHAT TO DO

- Formulate a food plan that provides at least 2,000 calories per person, per day, for no less than 90 days (longer if possible).

- Store an assortment of calorie-dense, shelf-stable foods that require no refrigeration, no cooking, and very little, if any, preparation. Simple heat-and-eat options are best.

- Maintain a variety of foods that you eat regularly, and rotate your supplies often to ensure freshness and to minimize spoilage and waste.

Quick Prep Tip

Proper planning, rotation, storage, and inspection of food packaging and containers can help reduce the chances of food-borne illness and can maximize your food storage efforts and dollars.

- Consider Meals-Ready-to-Eat (MREs), camping-style dehydrated foods, and long-term foods stored in number 10 cans and Mylar bags as a way of supplementing your supplies.

- Store all food products in cool, clean, dry conditions, away from heat, moisture, humidity, direct sunlight, and pests.

- Be mindful of food allergies and other medical issues when buying and storing food.

FOOD

Quick Prep Tip

Just-add-water, camping-style foods can provide an easy, lightweight, and convenient meal-in-a-pouch. These meals store well and rehydrate in minutes. The downside is that they can be expensive. Good option for a bug-out bag.

- If money is limited, start slowly, and incrementally add to your supplies.

- Avoid buying large quantities of long-term foods that you have not sampled for taste and digestibility.

- Take advantage of sales, coupons, and special offers to kick-start your food program.

- During a crisis avoid calling attention to yourself or your supplies by cooking outdoors—this is another reason why simple heat-and-eat options are best.

- Avoid any food in containers showing signs of rust, corrosion, damage to seal, or any cans that are dented, deformed, or bloated.

- Avoid any food that is discolored, mushy, moldy, or smells bad.

FOOD

WHAT TO GET

The following are examples of calorie-dense foods that store well and require little, if any, preparation:

- **Peanut butter**—Three-and-a-half tablespoons (100g) provides almost 600 calories, over 25g of protein, vitamins and minerals.

- **Almond butter**—Alternative if you don't like or are allergic to peanut butter.

- **Pasta**—Provides lots of carbohydrates for energy.

- **Pasta sauces**—Get a variety of flavors.

- **Canned macaroni and cheese, ravioli, spaghetti, tortellini, shells**—with beef, cheese, or other flavors.

- **Tuna**—Canned in water, one can (165g) has about 200 calories and over 42g of protein.

- **Sardines**—Canned-in-oil sardines have about 200 calories and about 23g of protein.

- **Chicken**—One can (140g) of chicken provides about 24g of protein and 140 calories.

- **Salmon**—One can (140g) of salmon provides about 85g of protein and 200 calories.

- **Canned meats**—Pork, beef, ham, turkey, etc. Get a variety.

- **Canned seafood**—Oysters, clams, mussels.

- **Canned soups**, stews, hash, and chili.

- **Canned vegetables**—Sweet peas, whole kernel corn, sweet corn, creamed corn, spinach, French-style beans, mushrooms.

Quick Prep Tip

Have at least two high-quality <u>manual</u> can openers, and several low-profile, self-contained heating options.

- **Rice**—One cup (195g) of cooked white rice has about 240 calories and over 4g of protein. (White rice stores better and keeps longer than other types of rice.)

- **Beans**—One cup (225g) of black beans has over 200 calories and 15g of protein. Canned beans can be warmed up and eaten right out of the can (black, red, white, navy, pinto).

- **Oats**—One cup (234g) of regular or quick oats has over 160 calories, 5.9g of protein, and is a concentrated source of fiber and nutrients.

- **Honey**—One ounce of honey has about 127 calories.

- **Evaporated, sweetened condensed, and instant powdered milk** are all good shelf-stable alternatives to regular milk.

- **Dark chocolate**—70 to 85 percent cacao solids, a (101g) bar has about 8g of protein and 600 calories.

- **Raisins, prunes, and other dried fruits**—portable, nutritious calories for energy.

- **Granola bars**—One bar usually provides 100+ calories, 5g protein, and 24g carbohydrates.

- **Protein bars**—Some protein bars have in excess of 500 calories, 45g of protein, and 50g of carbohydrates.

- **Nuts and seeds**—Almonds, cashews, walnuts, peanuts, and sunflower seeds contain about 200 calories per ounce.

- **Fruit in cans or jars**—Products packed in natural juices can also help with hydration.

- **Pancake mix and syrup**—Great comfort food and packed with tons of calories (two pancakes with syrup have over 500 calories).

- **Olive oil**—One tablespoon contains about 120 calories.

FOOD

- **Coconut oil** (extra virgin, unrefined) – One tablespoon contains about 125 calories.

- **Protein powder/meal replacement drinks**—One scoop (44g) of premium protein powder mixed with water provides 200 calories, and over 20g of protein, fiber, potassium, and carbohydrates.

- **Salt, pepper, flavorings, spices, dried herbs, and other common condiments** to prepare and flavor basic meals.

You can begin your food preparations by buying a few extra items each week. Over the next few months, your food stores will increase significantly. Test all new products before committing to any large purchases of any one item, and rotate your supplies on a regular basis.

Food Storage Conditions

Store all food products in cool, clean, dry conditions, away from heat, moisture, humidity, and direct sunlight (between 50-70 degrees Fahrenheit is a good range). Temperatures over 100 degrees are harmful to packaged and canned foods, and will radically reduce shelf life.

Quick Prep Tip

Drizzle a few teaspoons of olive, corn, canola, or vegetable oil on your survival meals as a calorie booster. These oils provide about 40-50 calories per teaspoon.

SURVIVAL AT A GLANCE

Expiration Dates and Food Storage

Food labeling dates are important and when used correctly, they can be a significant tool to assist in the management and rotation of your valuable supplies. The following are some of the most commonly used date-labeling terms, what they mean, and a short explanation of how to use them:

- **"Sell By":** This date usually lets the store know how long they should have the product on their shelves. This doesn't mean that the product will be unsafe to eat after the "Sell By" date. The date is a tool to help retailers rotate their inventory and displays. Under proper storage conditions, the product will probably be at its freshest if consumed by this date, but it will still be edible for a reasonable period of time after the "Sell By" date.

- **"Use By":** This is the manufacturer's recommended date of use to enjoy the product at the peak of freshness. This date may differ significantly for similar products, depending on the manufacturer.

- **"Best Before":** This date refers only to quality—it is not an indicator of safety. It's a suggested date to use the product at the best quality and flavor. Depending on storage conditions, many products will retain flavor, freshness, and quality far beyond this date.

BEST IF USED BY:

DEC 11 2013
1345 425 18:53 3

TP 30732001

There are many other date-labeling terms in use, and the laws governing manufacturer requirements differ from state to state. The actual meaning of each term will vary depending on who makes the product and where it's sold. Knowing what these dates mean and how to use them can be very useful in managing your food supplies to the fullest potential.

Quick Prep Tip

Meals-Ready-to-Eat (MREs) are a complete self-contained meal used by the military. MREs pack lots of calories and nutrition in a convenient pre-cooked package and have an estimated five-year shelf life (some even longer).

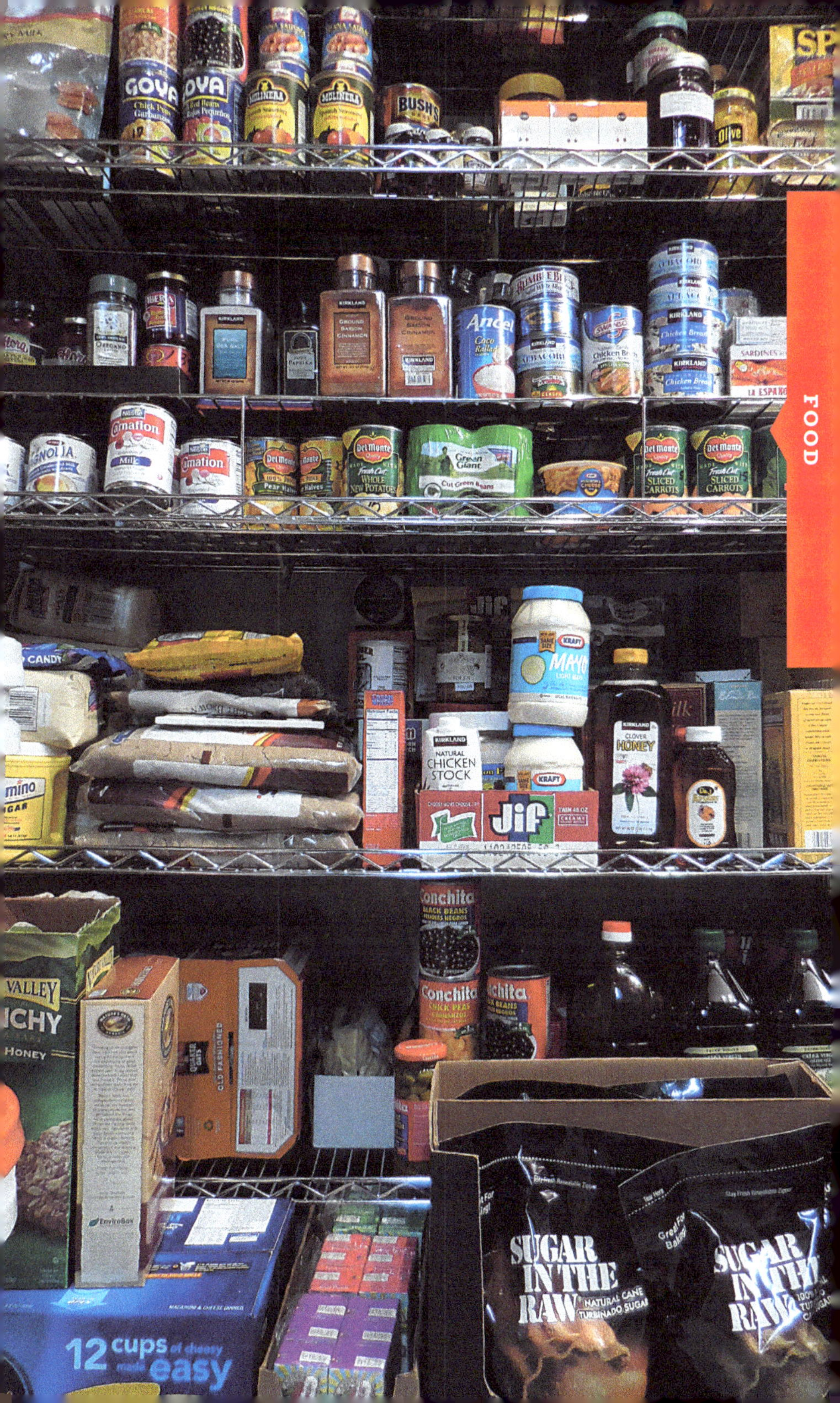
GOYA
Chick Peas
Garbanzos
GOYA
Red Beans
MOLINERA
MOLINERA
BUSH'S
Olive
KIRKLAND
Ground Saigon Cinnamon
Ancel
Coco Rallado
BUMBLE BEE
ALBACORE
Swanson
Chicken Breast
KIRKLAND
Chicken Breast
SARDINES
LA ESPAÑOLA
Carnation
Milk
Del Monte
Del Monte
Whole New Potatoes
Green Giant
Cut Green Beans
Del Monte
Sliced Carrots
Del Monte
Sliced Carrots
CANDY
KIRKLAND
Natural Chicken Stock
KRAFT
MAYO
Light Mayo
KRAFT
Jif
KIRKLAND
Clover Honey
Conchita
Black Beans
Conchita
Chick Peas
Garbanzos
Old Fashioned
12 cups of cheesy made easy
SUGAR IN THE RAW
Natural Cane Turbinado Sugar
SUGAR IN THE RAW

FOOD

WATER AND HYDRATION

WHAT TO KNOW

- Water is a top survival priority, second only to security and self-defense. Most people will not survive for more than three days without water.

- After a disaster, the public water supply may be unsafe or completely unavailable.

- Adequate hydration is essential to maintaining your ability to function; climate, environment, illness, and heavy exertion will all affect water intake requirements.

- Even crystal clear water may contain waterborne pathogens that can make you very sick. (All water is considered suspect until it has been disinfected.)

- Suspect water must always be disinfected before it is safe to drink. (Never use suspect water to brush your teeth; prepare food; wash pots, pans, or dishes; or to bathe.)

- Water can be disinfected by killing any organic, living, waterborne pathogens.

- The disinfection methods in this guide will not remove pollution or other chemical contaminants commonly found in many urban water sources.

- Dehydration occurs when you lose more water than you take in, resulting in your body not having enough fluids to function.

- Dehydration can be extremely dangerous; the safest approach is to prevent it by drinking enough water.

Never Be Without W...

Wa
emer

Stores up to
Fresh

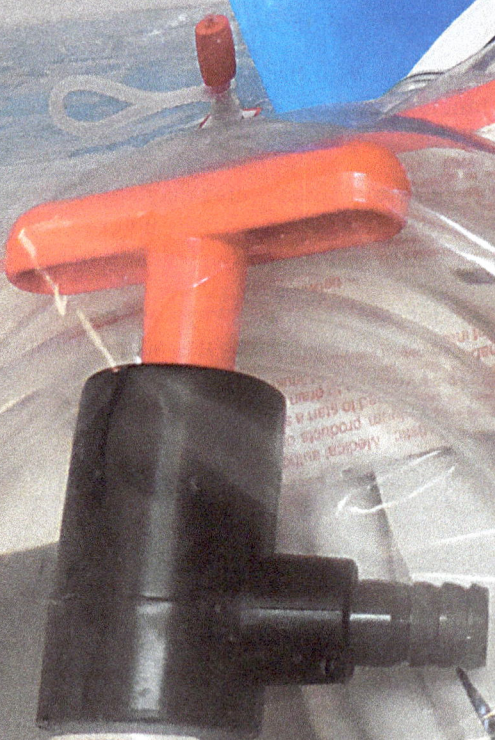

AZARD 10 PC
U.S. at. No.
4.3 1,826
ply
m & Check Pump's
s to Pumped
to Prevent
s Explosive
us Only
mical Equipment
ng

MINI

WATER FILTRATION SYSTEM

SAWYER

Filter up to
100,000
GALLONS from
freshwater
lakes, rivers,
or streams.

OB

r storage

ons of
Water

BOAT & CAMPER

CONSTRUCTED WITH · FABRICADA CON

REFLEX MESH

Eliminates kinks
Evita que se produzcan pliegues

DRINKING
WATER SAFE
APTA PARA
AGUA POTABLE

LEAD

LEAD-FREE
RoHS standards rest
Lead-free Cumple c
RoHS en la que refl
contenido de plom

EVERK

STRAIGHTENING HOS
QUE SE ENDEREZA AU

EED NOT TO KINK
OS QUE NO SE PLIEGA

menos de 0,1
géneo.

REVERSE S

Filtre à Eau Personnel

• Flow rate:
• 99.9999% de bacterias transportadas (bacteri pas
• 99.9% de p

Personal Water Filter

• Filters a minimum of 1,000 liters (264 gallons)
• Removes up to
• >99.9999% of waterborne bacteria (Giardia, Cryptosporidium)
• >99.9% of waterborne protozoan cysts
• Reduces turbidity by filtering particles to 0.2 microns
• Contains no chemicals

LifeStraw®

by VESTERGAARD

www.buylifestraw.com

WATER AND HYDRATION

- Consume plenty of water before, during, and after you are active. Don't wait until you're thirsty to start drinking water.

- The risk of becoming dehydrated is especially high during hot weather, heavy exertion, sweating, vomiting/diarrhea, or other illness.

- Drinking water is not enough—you must also maintain appropriate levels of essential minerals (electrolytes).

- Avoid eating heavy meals if water is in short supply, especially high-fat and protein-rich foods. These foods require a lot of water to digest. Instead, eat foods high in water content (i.e., fruits, vegetables, etc.).

- During a crisis, no water should be wasted. Recycle non-potable water for other uses. (Recycled water can still be used to flush toilets, for example.)

WHAT TO DO

- Store a minimum 30-day supply of emergency, short-term, bottled or tap water in water-safe containers—more if possible. (At least two gallons per person, per day, for drinking. Store extra for other uses.)

- Have an emergency long-term water plan with reliable access to alternate sources of clean water (i.e., a lake, stream, pool, water heater tank, etc.) See page 31.

- Have at least three different methods for disinfecting water—more if possible (chemical, heat, filtering, UV, SODIS, etc.).

- Store supplies to disinfect suspect water. This includes unscented household liquid bleach, 2 percent iodine, a deep pot with a lid to boil water, a large capacity water filter with extra filter elements, and supplies for solar and UV disinfection, etc. (Always use care when handling bleach to avoid injury.)

- Never underestimate the importance of water or the consequences of failing to have a viable water plan.

WHAT TO GET

- **Bottled water.** Store a minimum 30-day supply of bottled water (no less than two gallons per person, per day).

- **Water-safe containers.** Use food-safe containers that are BPA free to store water.

- **Water-safe hose** (usually white in color). Made with FDA-approved materials that are safe for drinking water.

- **Chlorine bleach** (unscented).

- **Plastic funnels** (different sizes and styles).

- **Manual water pump(s).** Have at least two, and use for drinking water only.

- **Tincture of iodine, 2 percent** and **povidone-iodine solution, 10 percent.**

- **Eye droppers** (store at least half a dozen).

- **Coffee filters,** to pre-filter water.

- **Large capacity water filter(s)** with **extra elements/filters.**

- **Small, portable water filter(s)** for when you're on-the-move.

- **Quart- and gallon-size plastic storage/freezer bags.**

Quick Prep Tip

Coconut water naturally contains essential electrolytes and more potassium than a banana. It's a natural way to stay hydrated and replenish lost electrolytes.

WATER AND HYDRATION

Quick Prep Tip

Our bodies sweat to regulate core temperature. However, sweating also causes the body to lose electrolytes.

SURVIVAL AT A GLANCE

CLEAR WATER CAN BE MADE SAFE TO DRINK BY:

- *HEAT*—Boil water for at least two minutes. Set it aside to cool.

- *CHEMICALS (Bleach)*—Add 2-4 drops of chlorine beach for every U.S. quart and let it sit for at least 30-45 minutes.

- *CHEMICALS (Iodine)*—Add 5-10 drops of iodine, 2 percent solution, for every quart and let it sit at least 30-45 minutes.

- *SOLAR RADIATION (Solar Disinfection or SODIS)*—Place water in a washed, clear plastic, one- or two-liter container and let it sit in full direct sunlight for a minimum of six hours. (Remove all labels from the plastic container to expose the water to the maximum amount of direct sunlight.)

- *FILTERING*—Many water filters will remove bacteria and parasites, but not viruses. New filter technology will remove bacteria and viruses. If in doubt, treat water with a disinfecting chemical after filtering. (Follow manufacturer's instructions for your filter.)

- *ULTRAVIOLET (UV) LIGHT*—Portable devices that deliver a measured dose of UV light to disinfect clear water. (Follow manufacturer's instructions for your UV unit.)

Never pour disinfected water back into a container that previously held the suspect water. The container must also be disinfected before you drink water out of it.

NOTE: *Always let cloudy or turbid water sit for about 30 minutes to allow sediments to settle at the bottom of the container before treating or filtering. Run the resulting water through a clean cotton cloth or a coffee filter to remove any additional debris. Repeat as necessary until water runs clear, then treat.*

ALTERNATE EMERGENCY WATER SOURCES

Stored water is your first line of water defense during any emergency, but you must also have a long-term plan in the event that your stored supplies run out or are somehow compromised. Consider alternate water sources your plan "B."

Most Common Sources of Emergency Water:

• **Rainwater**—Collected, disinfected, and stored in water-safe containers. Take steps to avoid contamination from animals, insects, and other environmental sources.

• **Melting ice or snow**—Can be a labor-intensive process, requiring a fuel-dependent heat source.

• **Pond, river, or stream**—Must be safely carried and treated, can become extremely labor intensive.

• **Pool water**—Unless it's really over chlorinated or somehow contaminated, pool water will usually be safe to drink in small quantities. Avoid consuming large quantities if unsure. (Pool water may also be exposed to other environmental contaminants which may make it unsafe.) Always exercise caution.

• **Spa or hot tub**—Probably won't taste all that good, but can be used as a last resort, again in small quantities.

WATER AND HYDRATION

WATER AND HYDRATION

- **Water heater tank**—A typical water heater can hold 50 gallons or more. Avoid water that contains rust, dirt, or that has a foul odor.

- **Toilet tank**—Water from the tank is usually safe, if there are no chemical additives. Never drink water from the bowl.

- **Water trapped in household plumbing**—Open faucet at lowest point of the dwelling, and let the water in the plumbing drain out. Turn off water main at first sign of contamination or other problems with the water supply.

- **Liquid from canned fruit and vegetables** is a good source of hydration.

- **Melted ice from freezer**—Plastic containers of frozen water serve the dual purpose of keeping the freezer cold during a power outage and of providing additional drinking water once the ice melts.

NOTE: *Never consume or use water that has an unusual smell, color, or taste. Suspect water must always be treated. All water is considered suspect until disinfected. Your first choice should always be to store enough safe water far in advance of any disaster.*

Quick Prep Tip

Water that is not safe to drink can still be used for other purposes: to flush toilets or to rinse five-gallon buckets that have been used to collect or dispose of waste, for example.

Dehydration and Electrolytes:

Water is a critical element that our bodies need to function properly. Dehydration occurs when the amount of water leaving the body exceeds the amount of water consumed. This is common during high temperatures, heavy exertion, and illness. In addition to drinking water, you must also maintain appropriate levels of essential minerals.

Dehydration is extremely dangerous and can quickly overtake even the strongest, most physically fit person. The very young and the elderly are at the highest risk. Avoiding dehydration will always be better than struggling to treat it "after-the-fact." Symptoms of dehydration may include:

WATER AND HYDRATION

Mild to Moderate Dehydration:

Headache

Confusion

Thirst

General discomfort

Dizziness and/or fainting

Dry mouth

Decreased urine output

No tears when crying

Constipation

Muscle cramping

Elevated body temperatures

Severe Dehydration:

Extreme thirst

Rapid breathing and heartbeat

Little or no urine, or dark urine

Decreased blood pressure

Very dry mouth

No tears when crying

Fever

Irritability or confusion

Sunken eyes

Staying well hydrated is crucial and should be a top priority. NEVER neglect water.

SURVIVAL AT A GLANCE

Simple Homemade Electrolyte Replacement Drink

This easy-to-prepare drink will replace electrolytes and trace minerals lost during heavy exertion or when you become dehydrated. An electrolyte deficiency can cause muscle and abdominal cramps, dizziness, nausea, and confusion. Make your own electrolyte replacement drink with healthier, more effective natural ingredients that are easily absorbed by the body (and it saves you money). It's easy:

Ingredients:

1 quart of clean disinfected water.

1 cup freshly squeezed orange juice (substitute 1/3 cup orange juice concentrate if fresh is unavailable).

½ freshly squeezed lemon/lime juice (substitute 8 teaspoons of lemon/lime juice concentrate if fresh is unavailable).

1/3 cup of honey (substitute 1/3 cup of organic/raw unbleached sugar if honey is unavailable).

1/2 teaspoon of sea salt.

Directions:

Mix salt and honey (or sugar) in one (1) cup of room temperature water. Add remaining water and mix well. If possible, cool and drink as needed. (Cool fluids are more quickly and effectively absorbed by the body than warm or cold fluids.)

PERSONAL SECURITY AND SELF-DEFENSE

WHAT TO KNOW

- The very first priority in any survival situation is security and self-defense.

- No amount of food, water, or other supplies will do you any good if you're dead or seriously injured.

- During (and especially after) any disaster, the police and other first responders will likely be overwhelmed and severely understaffed. You should not count on help from anyone outside your immediate group.

- Your main goal is to keep yourself and your family safe and secure.

- Personal security, self-defense skills, and preparations will give you options to protect yourself and your family.

- The best confrontation is the one that never happens. Whenever possible, avoid violent encounters, no matter how well prepared you may be.

- If you're able, flee the threat— get away as quickly and quietly as possible.

- If you can't avoid the threat, you must be ready, willing, and able to protect yourself and your family.

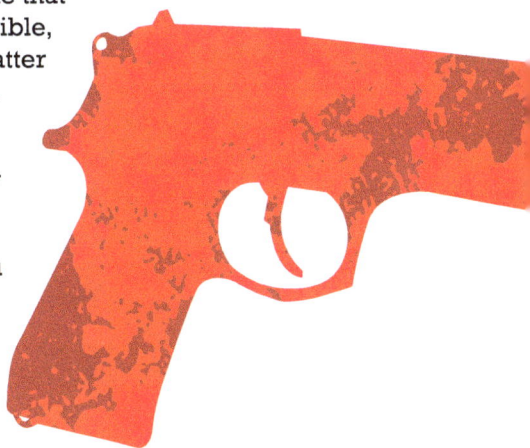

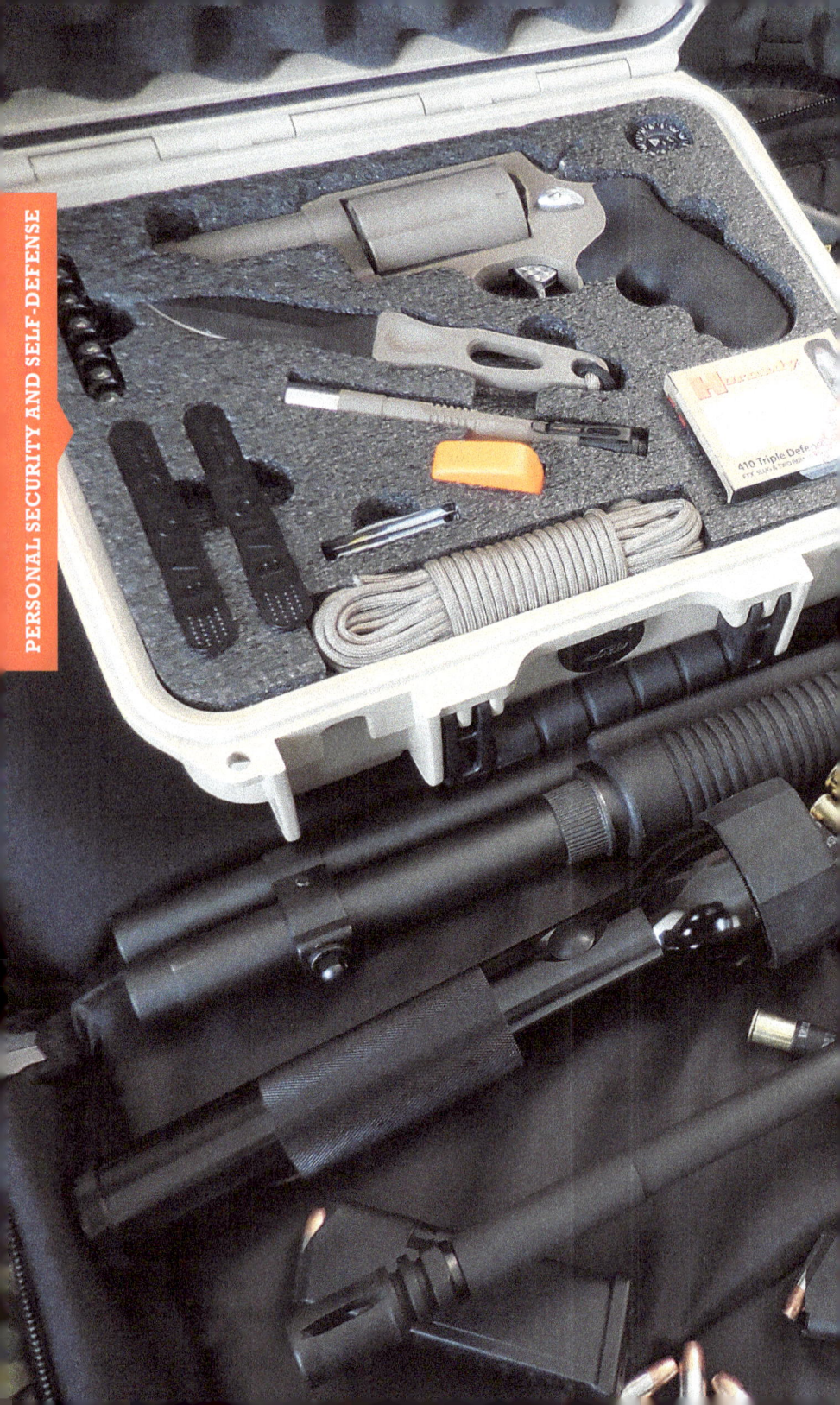

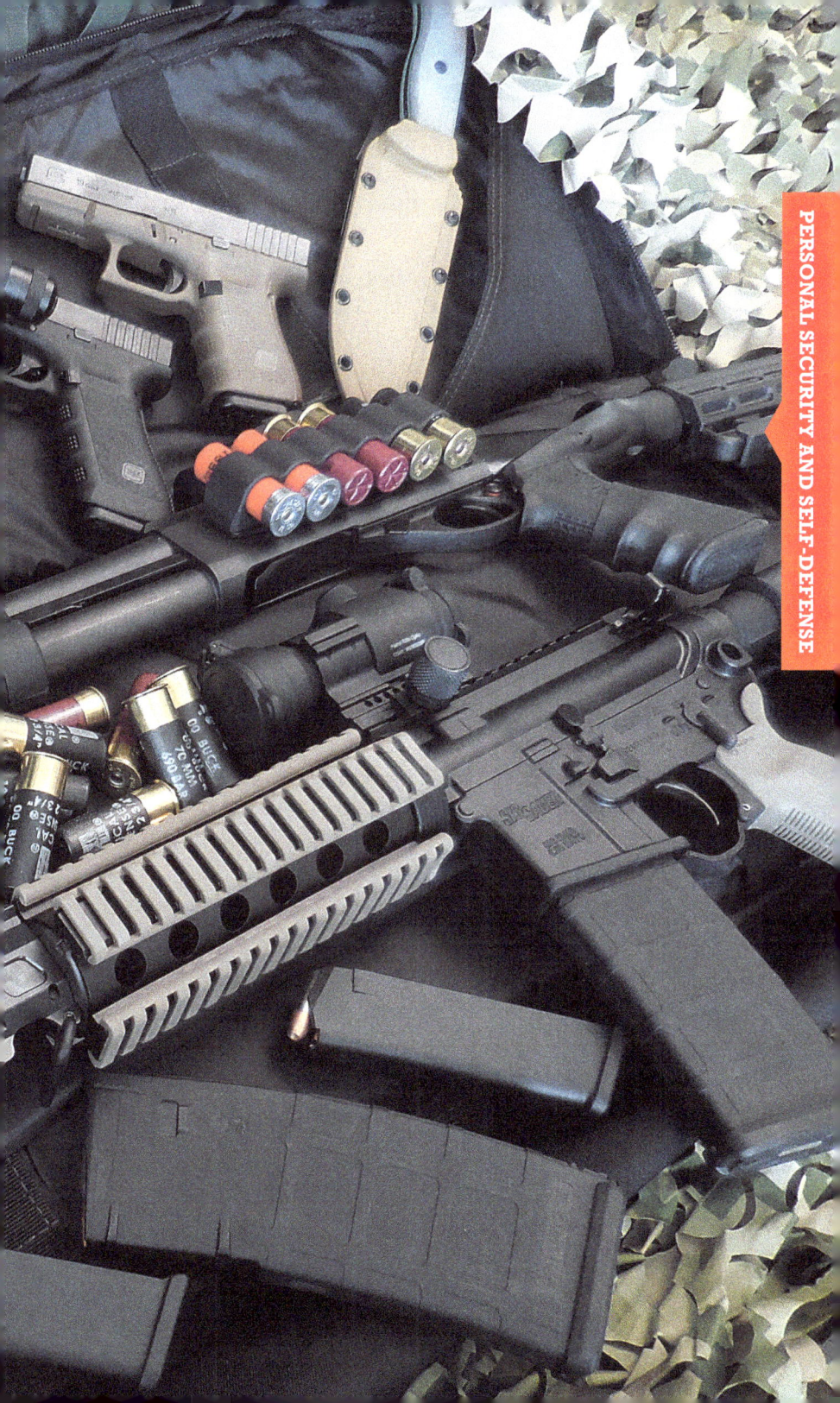

- If you must engage, have the means to address the threat quickly and decisively.

- A viable sheltering-in-place plan and supplies will allow you to avoid the chaos outside your front door and will complement your security plan.

- Violent crime is a major concern that can affect you at any time, not just during a disaster. You should always be keenly aware of your surroundings, prepared for the unexpected, and ready to defend yourself.

- It's important to have a viable plan and to communicate the details of that plan with all members of your group. Test your plan; if there are weaknesses, adjust accordingly.

WHAT TO DO

- Conduct realistic and practical self-defense assessments often; identify and address deficiencies in advance of any crisis.

- Develop and maintain a security and self-defense plan for your group—communicate all details, and ensure everyone understands their role and responsibilities.

- Maintain the proper mindset and avoid becoming a target/victim. Be aware of your surroundings, any potential threats, and always have a plan.

- Develop multiple levels of overlapping security and employ common sense.

- Avoid confrontations whenever possible.

- If you are unable to flee a threat, have the means and the mindset to decisively neutralize your opponent and end the fight quickly.

- Harden the perimeter, doors, and windows of your home against intruders.

- Install a security system, cameras, and early warning systems to alert you to potential dangers and any breach in security.

- Have sufficient supplies to quietly shelter-in-place for an extended period of time.

- During a crisis, maintain heightened security. Don't bring anyone into your home. If you must engage, do so outside. Desperate people will often do desperate things—don't take unnecessary chances.

- Avoid displaying lights at night. If the power is out, lights will announce to the world that you have supplies or at the very least, qualify you as a target of interest.

- Don't engage strangers, no matter how pathetic they may seem.

- Keep a low profile and avoid drawing attention to yourself or your group.

- Get the proper training, develop your skills, and have the tools to defend against threats.

- Maintain a high level of physical strength, endurance, and self-defense skills.

Quick Prep Tip

Set up a small "safe" room in your house for emergency situations. This is the shelter of last resort during severe weather or a home invasion.

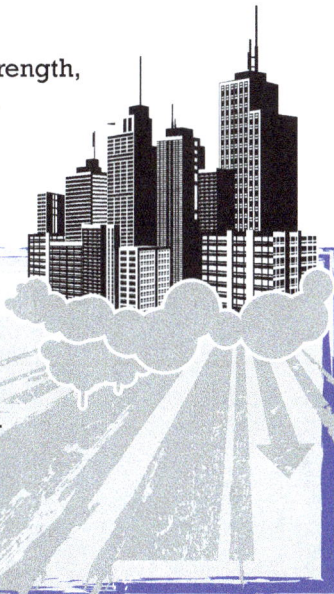

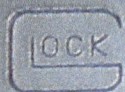

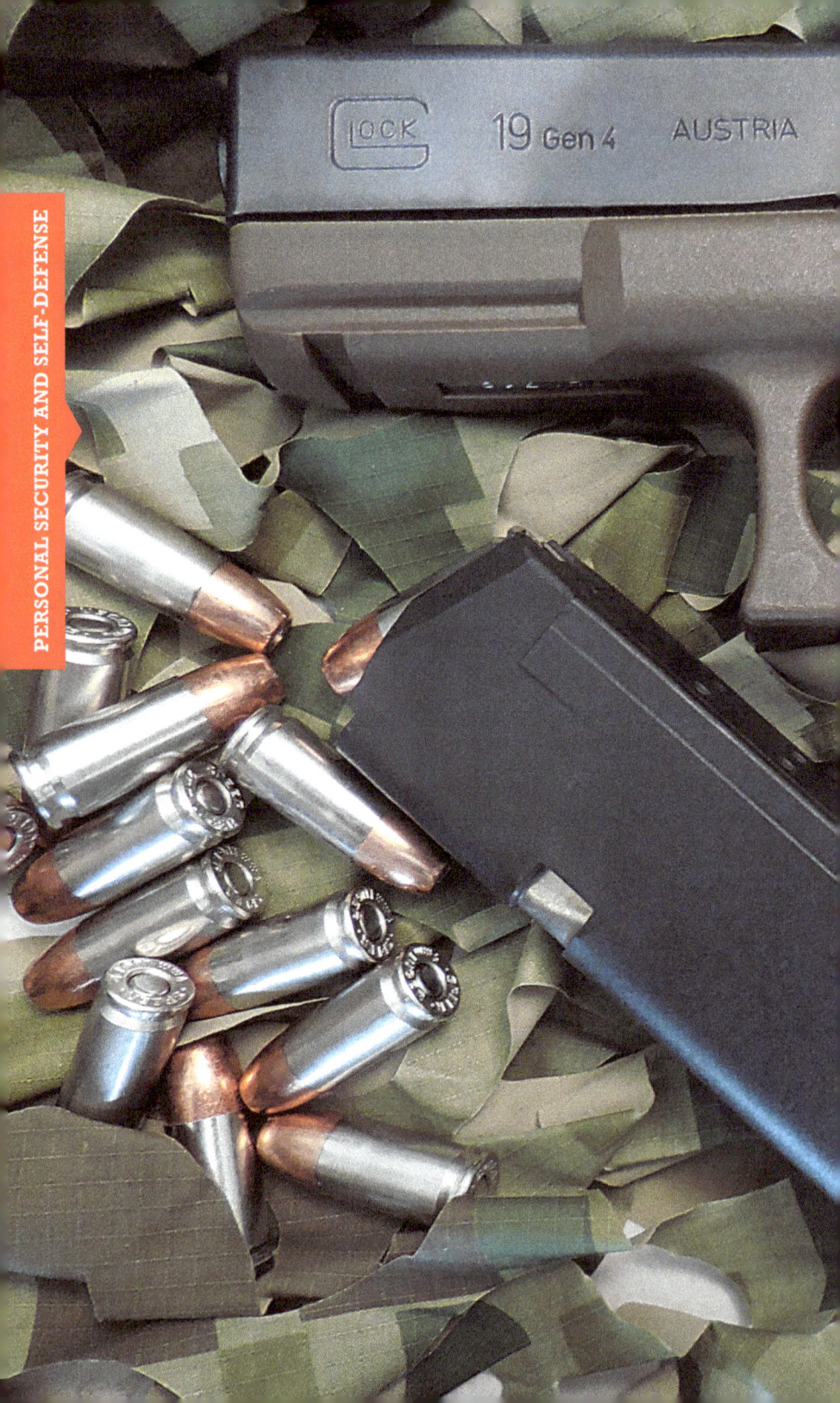

9×19

GLOCK

PERSONAL SECURITY AND SELF-DEFENSE

WHAT TO GET

- **Heavy-duty metal or solid-core wood doors**—For all exterior entrances, and any doorways leading to a bedroom or "safe" area within your house.

- **Door security hardware**—Deadbolts, latch bolt protectors, reinforced strike plates, and safety bars.

- **Impact resistant windows**—Laminated glass, engineered to stay in one piece and protect against severe weather or break-ins.

- **Security window film**—Extra strong, tear-resistant, safety film that protects windows from break-ins and severe weather by holding glass together if the window is broken. (Will not stop determined intruders, but will slow them down and give you time to escape, retreat, or arm yourself.)

- **Alarm system**—Sensors on all doors and windows, motion, smoke and broken glass detectors, panic buttons, and interior- and exterior-mounted sirens with LED indicators.

- **Fire extinguishers and smoke detectors**—Fire is a huge safety concern before, during, and after any disaster.

- **Security cameras**—With a DVR recorder and infrared night capabilities.

- **Firearms and a generous supply of defensive ammunition.**

- **Body armor** for all members of your group.

Quick Prep Tip

If you decide to use firearms for self-defense and protection, get the proper training. Know and follow the applicable laws in your jurisdiction.

Quick Prep Tip

Maintain the proper mindset and situational awareness to avoid becoming a victim.

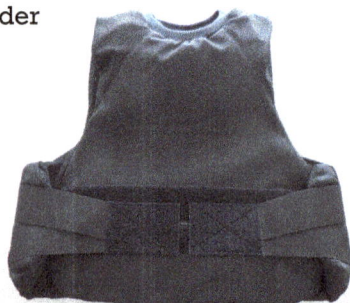

- **Firearms training** from qualified instructors and plenty of quality **practice**.

- **A safe** or other secure storage compartment for all firearms.

- **Less lethal defensive weapons**—Baton, pepper spray, stun gun, baseball bat, crow bar, etc. (Far less effective than firearms in a self-defense situation, but better than nothing.)

- **Adequate supplies of food, water, medical supplies, etc.** to avoid going out during a crisis, at least until the worst is over.

SURVIVAL AT A GLANCE

CHOOSING A SELF-DEFENSE FIREARM:

- **Price:** Firearms are not inexpensive; ammunition costs can also add up quickly. Find a balance between affordability and effectiveness.

- **Size and configuration:** Is the weapon for home defense or for concealed carry? Larger handguns are usually easier to handle and shoot. Smaller handguns are more difficult to control, but easier to conceal and carry. There is no one-size-fits-all firearm; test out the different options and judge for yourself.

- **Caliber:** Most self-defense experts do not recommend anything smaller than a 9mm round for self-defense.

- **Selection:** Pick a firearm that is easy to train with and easy to learn to use.

- **Maintenance:** Choose a firearm that is easy to clean and maintain. Dirty firearms can be unsafe and are more likely to fail when you need them.

- **Options:** Select a firearm that offers a wide selection of parts, accessories, and options.

NOTE: There are many resources available on the subject of selecting a firearm for self-defense. It's not possible to cover all the necessary considerations in this guide. But you should take the time to familiarize yourself with the viable options, and choose what works best for you and your situation/ circumstances. The most important thing is to be able to defend yourself and your group/family.

Quick Prep Tip

You will need physical strength, endurance, self-defense skills, and the proper tools to protect yourself and your family. Stay physically active and learn basic self-defense skills.

FIRST AID AND MEDICAL

WHAT TO KNOW

- Accidents and injuries will happen, and the only thing you can do is to be prepared.

- During a disaster, medical-care facilities and personnel (including hospital emergency rooms, doctors, healthcare workers and first responders) may be overwhelmed or completely unavailable.

- Every home needs a well-stocked first-aid kit and basic emergency medical supplies.

- A first-aid kit is designed to treat non-emergency situations that may not require a doctor or hospital (but that still need care to avoid complications), or to treat an emergency situation that requires immediate intervention until the person can be treated by a healthcare professional.

- Know the first-aid basics, and be prepared to assess and stabilize an injured person until help arrives.

- Avoiding an injury is always better than treating it. Don't take unnecessary risks and avert dangerous situations, especially during a crisis.

- Situational and safety awareness can help prevent many injuries. Be aware of your surroundings, and have a healthy respect for hazardous situations.

- Learn how to handle common injuries, including wounds, burns, cuts, trauma, etc.

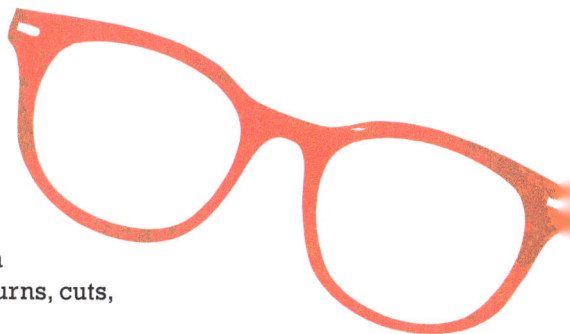

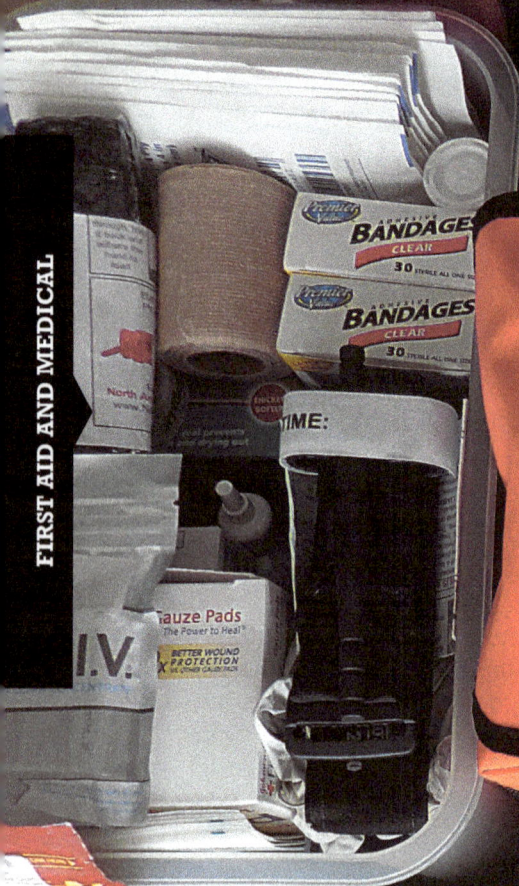
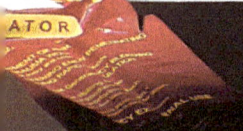
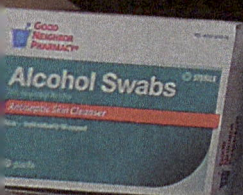
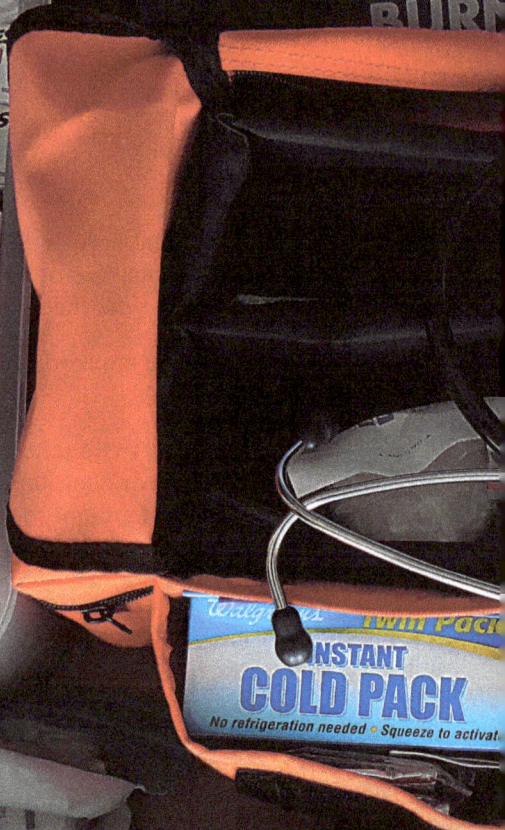
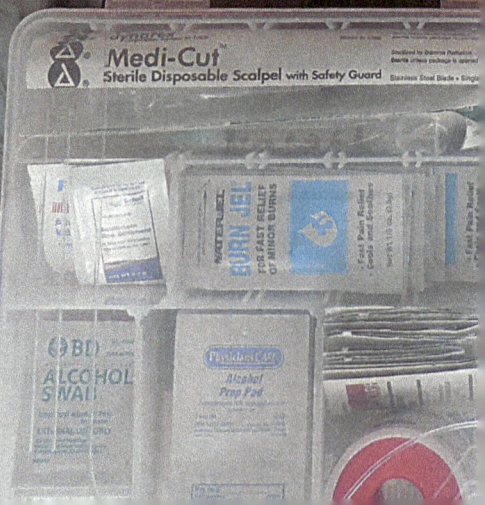

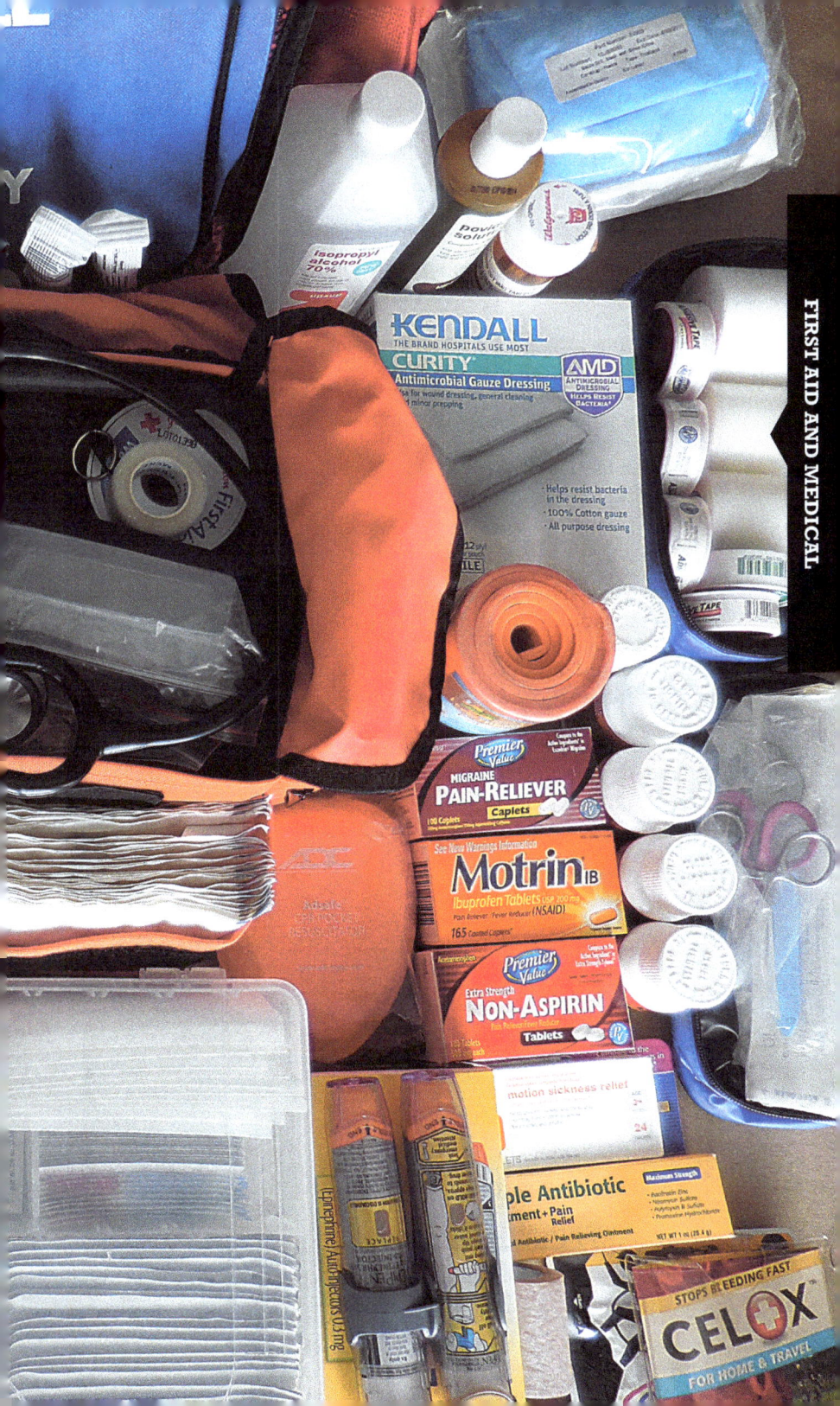

FIRST AID AND MEDICAL

WHAT TO DO

- Maintain well-stocked, use-specific, first-aid kit(s) and an ample inventory of emergency medical supplies/medications.

- Have a home first-aid kit for everyday use.

- Keep a basic kit and an expanded kit that remains untouched except for true emergency situations.

- Maintain a tactical trauma kit for extreme situations and life-threatening bleeds.

- Know what supplies are in your kits and how to use those supplies.

- Practice basic hygiene and sanitation techniques to reduce the risk of infection and the spread of disease.

- Rotate first-aid supplies and medications to ensure that you always have the freshest products available.

- Have a first-aid kit in your vehicle that's specifically adapted to where you live, work, and travel.

Quick Prep Tip

Making your own first-aid kit is easy, but remember that building and maintaining a functioning kit is an ongoing process requiring updating and rotation of supplies.

- Consult with your healthcare provider and ask for guidance on medications, precautions, or preparations you may need to make for your medical situation.

- Store at least a 90-day supply of medications and prescription drugs commonly used by you and your family.

- Have members of your group/household take a basic first-aid class.

- Have at least one person in your group trained to deal with pre-hospital trauma life support and violent trauma injuries.

- If you're unsure of what to do, it's often best not to do anything that may end up causing more harm.

- Maintain a strong and healthy body to help avoid medical issues during a crisis.

- Maintain dental health to avoid infections and other complications that can flare up during an emergency.

- Stay current on all recommended vaccinations.

- Take supplements to provide your body with necessary vitamins and minerals.

- Avoid high risk or dangerous situations that expose you to unnecessary hazards.

- Never take or give to another person any medication that was not specifically prescribed to that individual.

WHAT TO GET

You will need supplies for four different kits, as follows:

- **Basic**—Used for minor injuries and non-life-threatening situations that may require care to avoid complications.

FIRST AID AND MEDICAL

FIRST AID AND MEDICAL

- **Expanded**—Contains everything in the basic kit, plus more extensive supplies to treat emergency situations until the injured person can be taken to a doctor or hospital.

- **Tactical Trauma**—Contains everything in the expanded kit, plus supplies to treat serious trauma and life-threatening bleeds until medical help arrives or the person can be taken to a medical facility.

- **Vehicle Kit**—Contains everything in the basic kit, plus other supplies that you may need while on the road, specifically adapted to the types of roads and the terrain you typically travel.

Basic First Aid Kit

- **Tourniquet**—A compression device to apply pressure and control bleeding in the upper and lower extremities.

- **Hemostat granule wound treatment**—Helps stops bleeding.

- **Blood clotting granule applicator and plunger set.** Helps stop bleeding from a small, penetrating wound.

- **Gauze pads**—Large pads to clean, compress, and dress wounds.

- **Triangular bandage**—Multi-purpose bandage to compress various injuries; supports sprains or broken bones.

- **Tactical trauma dressing, Israeli-style bandage**—Applies direct pressure to stop bleeding in a hemorrhage wound.

- **Wound closure strips**—A sterile wound-closing system.

- **Transparent film**—Dressing designed for protecting skin and wound sites.

- **Nitrile exam gloves**—Disposable, latex-free gloves to minimize bacterial contamination when dressing wounds or tending to the injured (latex-free gloves avoid latex allergic reactions).

- **Adhesive bandages**—Selection of different sizes.

- **First-aid tape**—Waterproof first-aid tape in various sizes.

- **Elastic bandage (3-inch)**—Supports injured body parts and provides compression where needed.

- **Triple antibiotic ointment**—Treats and prevents infections in minor cuts, scrapes, or burns.

- **Burn treatment gel**—Soothes, cools, and temporarily relieves pain due to minor burns.

- **Povidone iodine (10% solution)**—Gold standard of external disinfectants. Kills germs in minor burns, cuts, and scrapes.

- **Alcohol prep pads**—Used to clean and sanitize, easy to store and use. Disposable.

- **CPR Face Shield**—Lets you give mouth-to-mouth resuscitation without the risk of contamination.

- **Ibuprofen**—Reduces pain and inflammation.

- **Acetaminophen**—Lowers fever and relieves pain.

- **Aspirin**—For a suspected heart attack.

- **Instant Cold Compress**—Back-up plan for pain and inflammation if no ice is available.

- **Hydrocodone**—This is for really serious pain – may be habit-forming and dangerous if misused. (You should consult with your doctor before taking any prescription medication, and you'll need a prescription).*

- **Ciprofloxacin**—A broad-spectrum antibiotic to attack bacteria. The big gun for bacterial infections. (You should consult with your doctor before taking any prescription medication, and you'll need a prescription).*

FIRST AID AND MEDICAL

51

- **Loperamide**—Stops diarrhea that can cause life-threatening dehydration.

- **Disposable Thermometers**—Sterile, single-use clinical thermometers that are lightweight, accurate, and disposable.

- **Portable Electrolyte Hydration**—Active hydration tablets that dissolve in water and are easy to use.

- **First-aid Accessories**—Flashlight with extra batteries, shears, bandage scissors, forceps.

Expanded First Aid Kit (beyond the Basic Kit)

- **IV fluids and needles** (different sizes)

- **Sutures** (different sizes)—have a variety

- **Needle holders, suture scissors, and forceps**

- **Antibiotics**—To treat bacterial infections. (You should consult with your doctor before taking any prescription medication; you'll need a prescription).*

- **Epinephrine injection**—Used to treat life-threatening allergic reactions caused by insect bites, foods, medications, latex etc. (You'll need a prescription, and you'll also need to know how to use it properly.)*

- **Blood pressure set**—Quality cuff and stethoscope.

- **Resuscitation bag**—To provide ventilation when a person's breathing is insufficient or has ceased.

- **Eye pads**—To bandage eye injuries.

- **Eye wash**—Sterile irrigating solution for emergency eye cleansing.

- **Activated charcoal**—To treat poisonings and intestinal gas.

- **Moleskin**—To cover and protect blisters and sensitive skin.

- **Berman Oral Airway Kit**—To keep airways open. Single use, latex-free.

- **Aluminum Splint**—Help support and immobilize injured limbs.

Tactical Trauma Kit

Maintain a tactical trauma kit for serious wounds or other life threatening bleeds.

- **Tourniquet**—A compression device to apply pressure and control bleeding in upper and lower extremities.

- **Hemostat granule wound treatment**—Helps stops bleeding.

- **Blood Clotting Granule Applicator and Plunger Set**—Helps stop bleeding from a small penetrating wound.

- **Gauze Pads (4X4-inch)**—Store an abundance of these.

- **Triangular Multi-Purpose Bandage.**

- **Nitrile Exam Gloves**—Disposable latex-free gloves.

- **Elastic Bandage (3-inch)**

- **Israeli Battle Bandage (4-inch)**

- **Chest Seal**—For the management of penetrating chest wounds.

Quick Prep Tip

Maintain several well-stocked first aid kits — Basic, Expanded, and Trauma-specific kits are best.

FIRST AID AND MEDICAL

Quick Prep Tip

Keep a minimum of a 60-90 day supply of all prescription medications that you or your family members routinely take.

SURVIVAL AT A GLANCE

The following is a list of some of the most common antibiotics:

- **Ciprofloxacin:** Used to treat or prevent anthrax, among other things.

- **Amoxicillin:** A penicillin antibiotic used to treat many different types of infections caused by bacteria.

- **Erythromycin:** Used to treat bronchitis, diphtheria, Legionnaire's disease, pertussis, pneumonia, rheumatic fever, venereal disease, ear, intestine, lung urinary tract, and skin infections. Sometimes used in penicillin-allergic patients instead of amoxicillin.

- **Co-Trimoxazole:** Eliminates bacteria that cause infections of the urinary tract, lungs, ears, and intestines (traveler's diarrhea).

- **Doxycycline:** Fights bacteria in the body. Used to treat pneumonia, Lyme disease, skin infections, anthrax, urinary tract infections, and to prevent malaria.

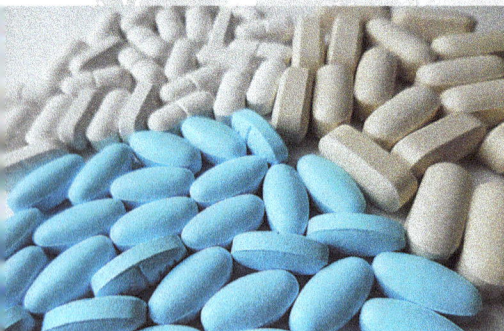

NOTE: Antibiotics may cause side effects and allergic reactions. To protect your health, only take antibiotics prescribed by your doctor and follow the instructions.

*NOTE: READ THIS – VERY IMPORTANT

Having medical supplies and medications, and using those supplies correctly, are two entirely different things. You should never take a prescription medication that has not been properly prescribed to you by a qualified medical professional. You should not take any medications that you are not familiar with before consulting with your doctor or a qualified health care professional. Some medications, including antibiotics, can have severe side effects and, in some people, can cause more harm than good. The unsupervised use of any prescription medication is extremely dangerous and can potentially be fatal. Talk to your doctor and find out what medication(s) he/she recommends that you keep on hand for your particular situation, and also talk to your doctor about the risks of using any of those medications for your condition(s). Find out if you have any allergies to any medications (for example, penicillin) and make sure that other members of your group or family know of your allergies in case you are injured and you can't communicate with your caregiver(s).

The information provided in this guide is provided for illustration purposes only and does not provide, nor is it intended to provide, medical or any other type of professional advice to any reader. Any use of the information contained in this book shall be solely at the reader's risk.

Quick Prep Tip

The supplies in a vehicle first-aid kit should be examined and rotated more frequently since these kits are often exposed to temperature extremes and humidity.

FIRST AID AND MEDICAL

HYGIENE & SANITATION

WHAT TO KNOW

- Sanitation is about properly disposing of trash and human waste, and maintaining a clean environment to minimize the chance of spreading contamination and disease.

- Lack of proper sanitation and hygiene can kill just as quickly as lack of food, water, or security.

- During a disaster, lack of clean water, solid waste retrieval, and general lack of proper sanitation, can render urban areas virtually uninhabitable.

- Proper planning and preparations can help keep you clean and healthy.

Quick Prep Tip

Nothing you can do will ever be 100 percent effective in preventing the spread of disease or contamination. But, simple precautions will minimize the chances of these conditions spreading among your group. Make sure to establish and clearly communicate these life-saving procedures to all the members of your group.

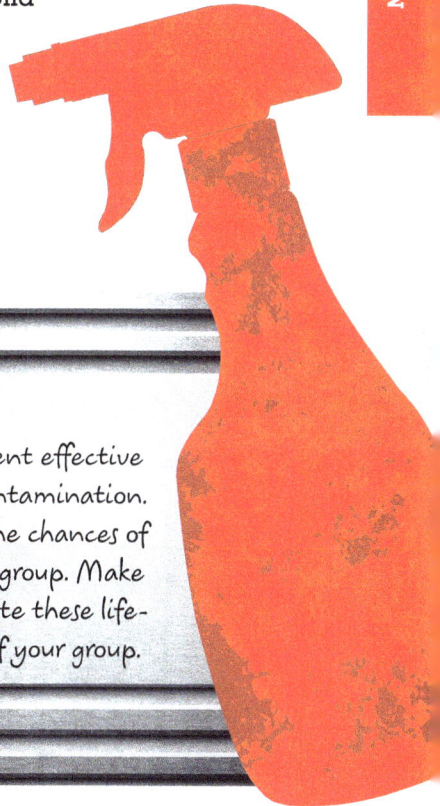

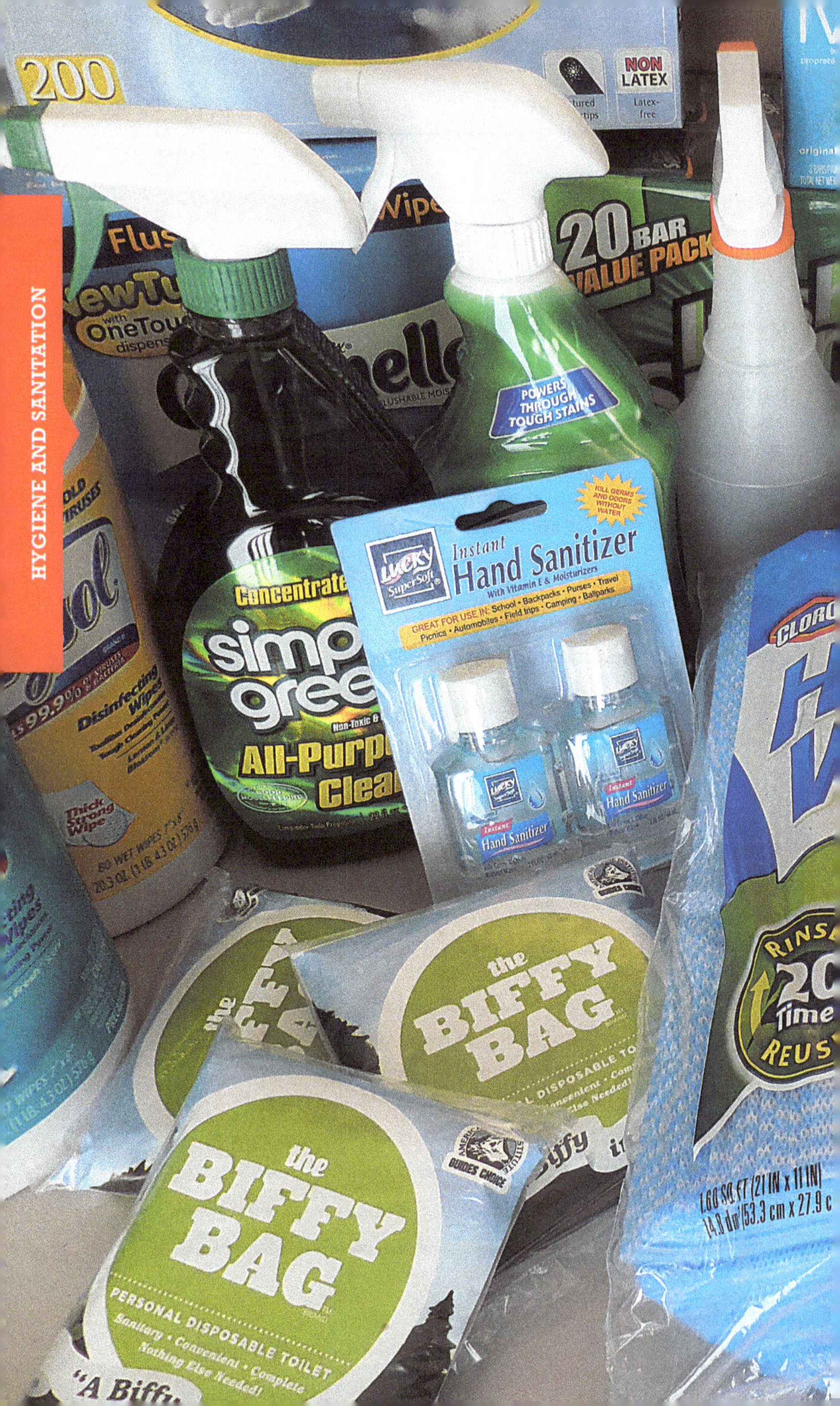
200
NON LATEX
Latex-free
20 BAR VALUE PACK
POWERS THROUGH TOUGH STAINS
Concentrate
simple green
All-Purpose Cleaner
KILL GERMS AND ODORS WITHOUT WATER
Instant Hand Sanitizer
With Vitamin E & Moisturizers
GREAT FOR USE IN: School • Backpacks • Purses • Travel
Picnics • Automobiles • Field trips • Camping • Ballparks
Hand Sanitizer
Disinfecting Wipes
99.9%
Thick Strong Wipe
80 WET WIPES
20.3 OZ (1 LB 4.3 OZ) 576g
the BIFFY BAG
PERSONAL DISPOSABLE TOILET
Sanitary • Convenient • Complete
Nothing Else Needed!
GUIDES CHOICE
CLOROX
RINSE 20 Times REUSE
1.60 SQ FT (21 IN x 11 IN)
14.9 dm² (53.3 cm x 27.9 c

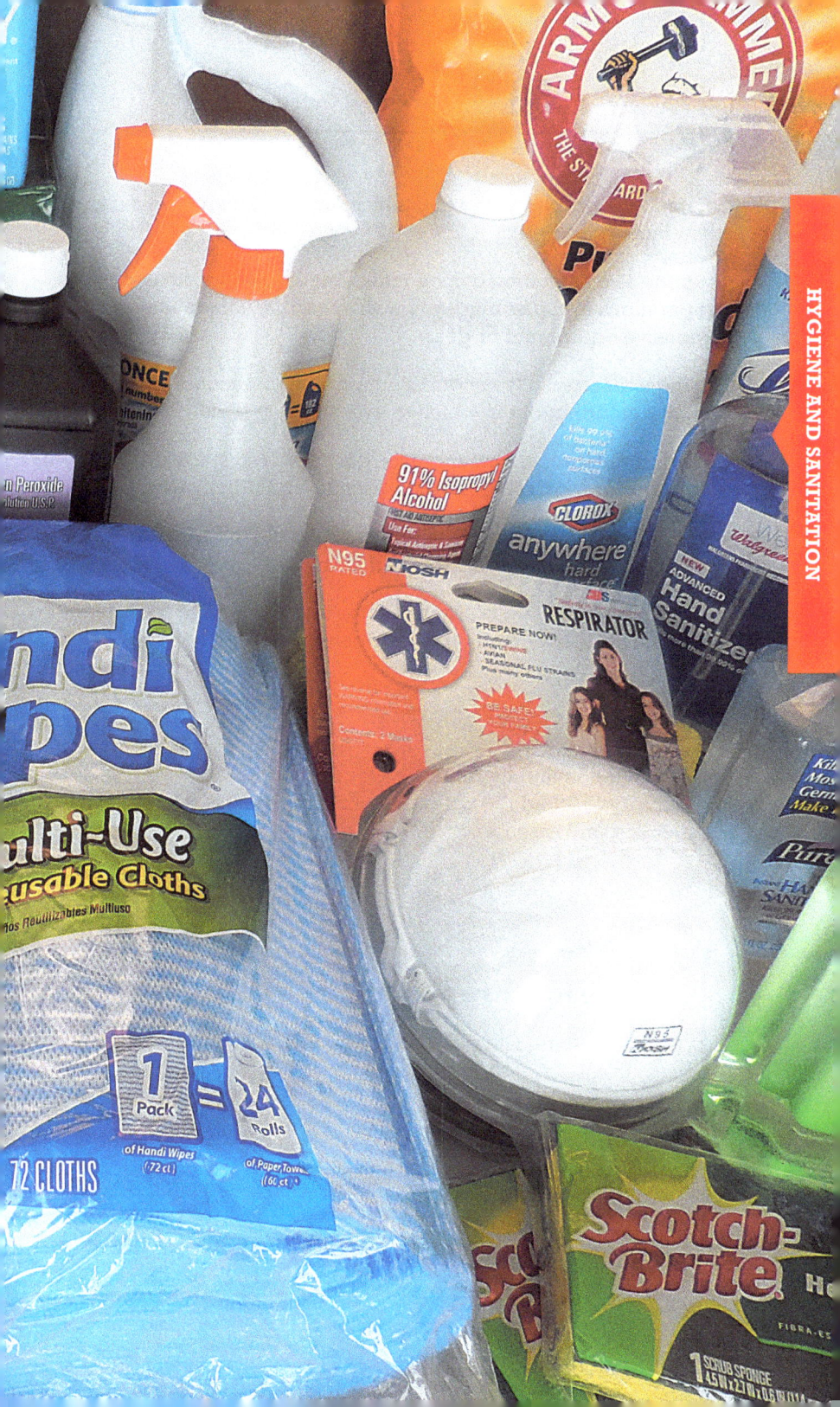

- Sanitation is probably one of the most neglected areas in survival planning.

- Hygiene and sanitation can be maintained with some basic preparations and planning; you won't need any complicated or expensive equipment or gear.

- During a disaster, it is especially important to maintain a clean and sanitary environment in which to live, sleep, and eat.

- The accumulation of human waste, garbage, and stagnant water will attract disease-carrying rodents, insects, and other pests.

- You'll need basic planning, supplies, and a clear understanding of how to avoid the situations that can harm you.

- Preventing a problem is always better than struggling to fix it after the fact. This is especially true with sanitation and hygiene.

WHAT TO DO

- Make sanitation and hygiene a top priority to avoid the spread of infection and disease.

Quick Prep Tip

Stock up on all the necessary supplies in advance. Most of these items are relatively inexpensive and non-perishable; your supplies will keep for many years if properly stored.

- Have a plan and supplies for efficiently getting rid of human waste and trash.

- Have supplies and a plan for keeping clean with minimum amounts of water (or no water).

- Use plastic/paper disposable plates, cups, and utensils.

- Store toilet paper, paper towels, napkins, and tissues.

- Also store plastic garbage bags, 5-gallon plastic buckets with lids, antibacterial wipes/gels/soaps, and personal hygiene products.

- Prepare a solution of three parts water mixed with one part household bleach, and put it in a spray bottle for sanitizing and disinfecting hands.

- Drink bottled water whenever possible.

- Always disinfect suspect water before using it. (All water is suspect until disinfected.)

- Use disinfected water to prepare food.

- Use disinfected water to wash items used in eating or preparing food. Better yet, use disposable cups, plates, etc.

- Wash hands with soap and disinfected water as often as possible, especially after using the toilet or after taking care of someone who has diarrhea or is ill.

- Always store the clearly marked disinfected water in a clean, covered container to prevent recontamination.

- Use protective clothing, gloves, and a surgical mask when treating someone who has diarrhea, or who is known or suspected to be ill. (The mask is intended to stop you from inadvertently touching your mouth or face with dirty hands.)

- Use protective clothing, gloves, and a surgical mask when disposing of feces or cleaning out your toilet facilities.

HYGIENE AND SANITATION

- Use plastic bags to hold feces/diapers, and dispose of all such plastic bags in plastic or metal garbage cans as far away as possible from your food, water, and living area.

WHAT TO GET

Here's a list of basic supplies. Adapt these supplies to your individual needs and circumstances. Remember, this is just a starting point.

- **5-gallon buckets and lids**—These buckets have many uses and are extremely durable.

- **Household bleach** (unscented).

- **Spray bottles** (various sizes).

- **Anti-bacterial soap**—Liquid and bars.

- **Anti-bacterial gels** and hand sanitizers.

- **Anti-bacterial wipes.**

- **Disinfecting sprays**—For odor control and surface disinfection.

- **Household cleaning products**—Assortment of the most commonly used products.

- **Alcohol and alcohol wipes**—For sanitation and disinfection.

- **Heavy-duty plastic garbage bags** (various sizes).

- **Portable/camping style toilets.**

- **Face masks**—High quality N95 masks.

- **Nitrile gloves**—Large assortment of different sizes.

- **Eye shield/protection**—To protect against splatter.

- **Toilet paper, paper towels, napkins.**

- **Disposable plastic or paper plates and cups.**

- **Disposable plastic forks, spoons, knives, and serving utensils.**

- **Baking soda**—Deodorizer, cleaner, fire extinguisher, fruit and vegetable scrub.

- **White vinegar**—Eliminates germs and odors; used as a cleaner.

- **Cat litter**—To cover human waste in portable or makeshift toilets.

SURVIVAL AT A GLANCE

Hand Washing with Minimum Water:

You'll need to keep your hands clean to prevent the spread of disease and infection, but washing your hands with suspect water will only encourage the spread of any contaminants. Here are some tips to help you keep your hands clean, using the minimum amount of your precious disinfected water:

- Use an alcohol gel or some other form of antimicrobial hand sanitizer; these products can be effective in the short term.

- Wash your hands using a small amount of water and soap in a bucket or sink. Rinse in another receptacle, again using a small amount of clean water, then dry off with a paper towel. (Do not handle the water containers with dirty hands. Instead, have someone in your group pour the clean water over your hands.)

- Prepare a solution of three parts clean water and one part unscented chlorine bleach, and pour the solution into a spray bottle. Have another person spray your hands while you rub them together. Rinse with clean water, and air dry or use a clean paper towel.

GETTING OUT FAST
(BUGGING OUT)

WHAT TO KNOW

- Bugging out is the act of leaving your present location in a very big hurry and relocating to a safer, more secure location, typically with a pre-packed bug-out bag (BOB).

- Bugging out can be extremely dangerous and should only be considered as a last resort. Your home will usually be the safest place to be after a disaster.

- Bugging out requires supplies, a plan, a destination, an alternate plan and destination, and the means to get you there safely.

- At times, it may be necessary to bug out, even if you don't have a place to go or a plan. If you lose your home to fire, destruction, criminals, etc., you may have to leave for safety reasons. This is why you need a plan, back-up plans, supplies, and a well-stocked BOB, even if you don't plan on bugging out.

- The majority of the population will be completely unprepared to deal with any disaster lasting more than a few days. Many will attempt to flee urban areas, but they will have no planned destination and few, if any, supplies.

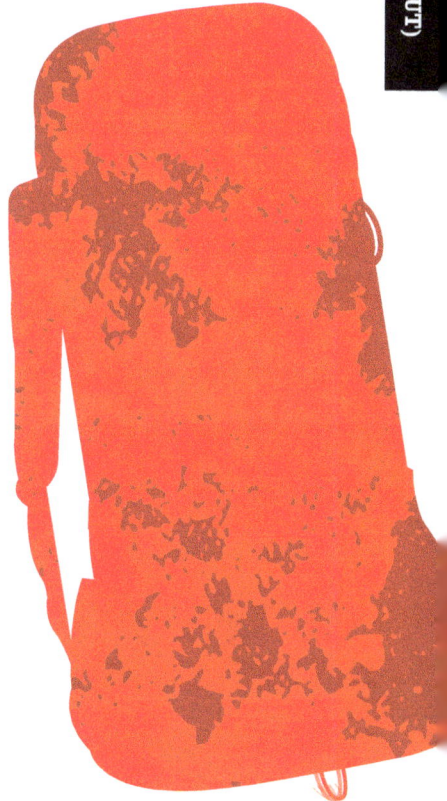

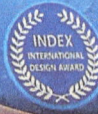
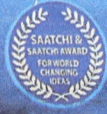

GETTING OUT FAST (BUGGING OUT)

estraw by VESTERGAARD

EESE TORTELLINI IN TOMATO SAUCE

ATURE VALLEY.
CRUNCHY
ts 'n Honey
16g of whole grain

I WITH BEANS

POTABLE AQUA

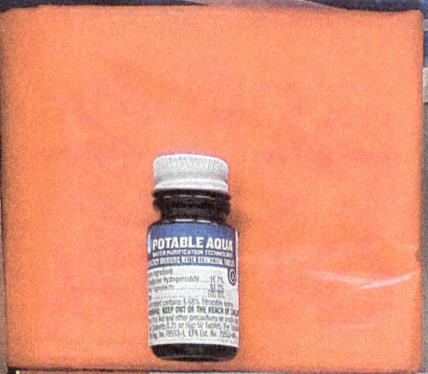

+ EYESHIELD
SINGLE USE
CHILD
1 Mask for Ages 5+

+ EYESHIELD
SINGLE USE
ADULT
1 Mask

ReadiMask

Adhesive-Sealing
Particle Mask
with Anti-Fog Eyeshield

MADE IN THE USA

ENHANCED PROTECTION IN HAZARDOUS AREAS
Complete Perimeter Seal   Hypoallergenic Medical Adhesive
Comfortable, Easy to Breathe   Eyeglasses Go Over Eyeshield

SUBSTANTIALLY PROTECTS AGAINST
FLU / VIRUS   MOLD   PEPPER SPRAY
BACTERIA   DUST   POLLUTION
SPORES   DEBRIS   SMOKE PARTICLES
ALLERGENS   HAZARDOUS PARTICLES

Sterling Foods
WHEAT SNACK BREAD

Sterling Foods
WHEAT SNACK BREAD

Pangea WORLD BAKERS
Brownie With Chocolate Chips

Pangea WORLD BAKERS
Brownie With Chocolate Chips

POWER HEAT
2-HOUR CHAFING DISH FUEL
Net Wt. 7 oz. (198g)

JetScream

Purell
INSTANT HAND SANITIZER
with Aloe
#1 DOCTOR

EMERGE

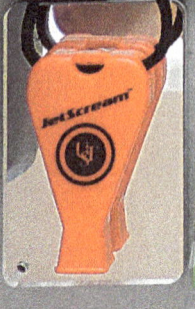
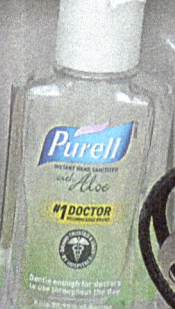
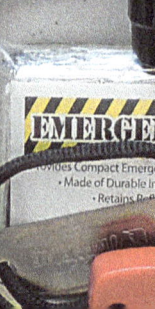

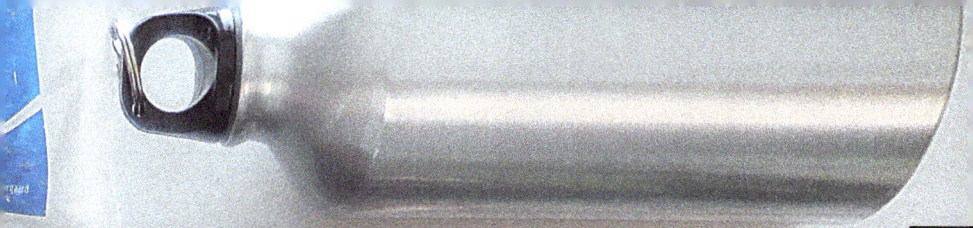

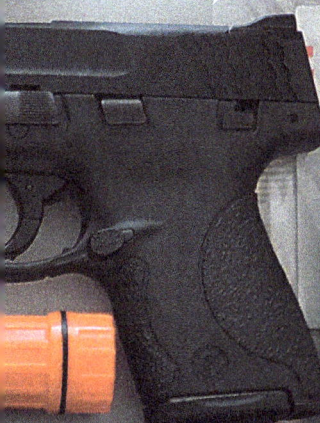
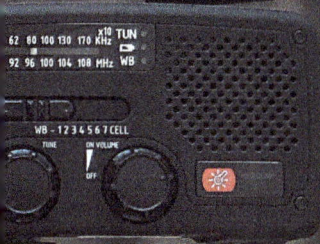
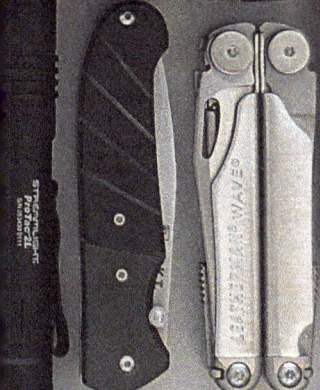
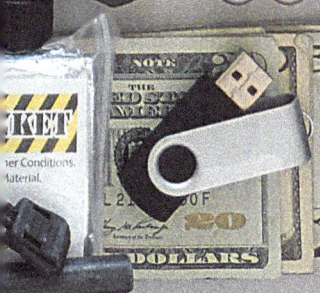
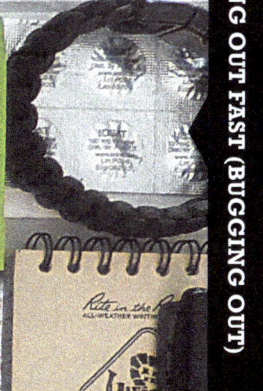

IOSAT

NDC 51803-001-

INDICATIONS:
THYROID BLOCKING IN A
RADIATION EMERGENCY ONLY

RAND M^cNALLY

streets of
Miami Metro

FEATURES
Full Street Index

COMMUNITIES
INCLUDED
Coral Gables

Emer
1,000
Vita
DIETARY SU
Tange
Flavored Fizzy Drin

Cottonelle
Fresh

Verizon
Prepaid Long Distan   ne Ca
Minutes NEVER
PINless Dialing & Expr
Great International Rates fro

zippo

Rechargeable
Prepaid Long Distance Phone Car

Scotch Super 88
Vinyl Electrical Tape
054G07-06143

5-hour
ENERGY
EXTRA
STRENGTH
SOUR APPLE

ACCEL
ADVANCED SPOR

EXTENDS ENDUR
SPEEDS MUSCLE
PROVIDES MORE

DOLLARS

- Most stores, gas stations, and banks will be overwhelmed by desperate people seeking food, water, gasoline, and cash in order to leave the area. Looters and criminals will quickly target the most vulnerable segments of the population.

- Roads, highways, and other transportation arteries will quickly become overwhelmed by unprecedented levels of traffic and abandoned vehicles.

WHAT TO DO

- Assess your vulnerabilities and options well in advance of any disaster.

- Formulate your plans, and always have back-up plans for leaving or staying.

- Make your own BOB (72-hour kit) and customize it to suit your particular needs and circumstances.

- Test your bug-out plans regularly. An untested plan is as good as no plan at all. If your plan fails during testing, you still have an opportunity to modify it.

- Review, rotate, and update the contents of your BOB regularly. Keep all supplies current.

- Have an established relationship and plans with people situated outside your community. Otherwise, don't expect a warm welcome when you show up unexpectedly after a disaster.

- Have a map of your intended bug-out route(s), marking locations of interest, including police/fire stations, hospitals, and water sources. (Also mark areas to avoid.)

- Learn how to navigate using a compass.

- Maintain at least one vehicle with a full tank of gas that's ready to go on a moment's notice. This vehicle must be mechanically sound and realistically capable of getting you to your intended destination.

- Establish and maintain reliable access to additional emergency fuel for your vehicle. Storing fuel can be dangerous. Only use containers approved by local, state, and federal authorities for storage and transportation, and always store your fuel in a well-ventilated area away from your home, heat, or direct sunlight. (Check local laws on how much fuel you can store.)

WHAT TO GET

- **A heavy-duty book bag** with sturdy padded straps. Avoid tactical or military looking bags. A black, average-looking bag will blend in with the crowd and is usually the best option.

- **Compass and map** of your expected travel area(s).

- **Lightweight energy food**, protein bars, MREs, snacks, hard candy, gum.

- **Bottled water, portable water filter(s), water purification tablets, iodine, and household liquid bleach.**

- **LED flashlight/headlamp with extra batteries, light sticks** (2-6).

- **Radio** (hand crank preferred) or with extra batteries.

GETTING OUT FAST (BUGGING OUT)

Quick Prep Tip

Cash is king. During a crisis, ATMs and credit card terminals may be down, and banks may be closed. Keep enough cash on hand to help get you out of town. (Small bills are best; spread your stash among different pockets, and keep some hidden in a travel-style waist wallet.)

GETTING OUT FAST (BUGGING OUT)

- **Cell phone and charger.**

- **First aid kit**—Small kit with a little of everything you may need.

- **Prescription medication** (no less than 72 hours, more if possible).

- **Masks (N95), nitrile gloves, eye and ear protection.**

- **Potassium iodide tablets** to protect your thyroid gland from radiation.

- **Moleskin**—To protect sensitive feet when walking long distances.

- **Sun screen and bug repellent.**

- **Multi-tool, large and small knifes, small scissors and a compact sharpener.**

- **Fire starter, waterproof matches, lighter(s).**

- **Soap, small hand towels, antibacterial gel, travel size roll of toilet paper, small supply of personal hygiene products.**

- **Petroleum jelly** (small tube) to protect skin and lips, start fires, and tool lubricant, etc.

- **Plastic tarp, rain poncho, bungee cord(s), Mylar blankets.**

- **Extra clothes, socks, hat, gloves, and walking shoes/boots.**

- **Cash** (small bills and some coins)—At least $250.00 to $500.00.

- **Heat source** (gel fuel style cans)—Small solid-fuel stove or candles.

- **Duct and electrical tape, re-sealable plastic bags, 550 Paracord (100').**

- **Firearms, extra magazines and ammunition, pepper spray, baton, etc.**

- **Water-resistant plastic storage bag** to keep copies of important documents (passport, driver's license, Social Security card, concealed weapons permit, etc.).

- **Flash drive** (password protected) containing scanned copies of important legal and financial documents.

- **List of contact information**, phone numbers, addresses, etc.

- **Pre-paid calling card** (in case your cell phone is lost/damaged or if service is down).

Adjust the contents of your bag to the anticipated weather conditions, time of year, and the terrain you will travel.

Quick Prep Tip

Don't over pack. Walking long distances with a heavy pack strapped to your back is extremely difficult. Pack your BOB with the essentials, and have a second bag with desirable, but not essential items. If you need to shed weight along the way, the second bag can be left behind, given away, or traded for other supplies.

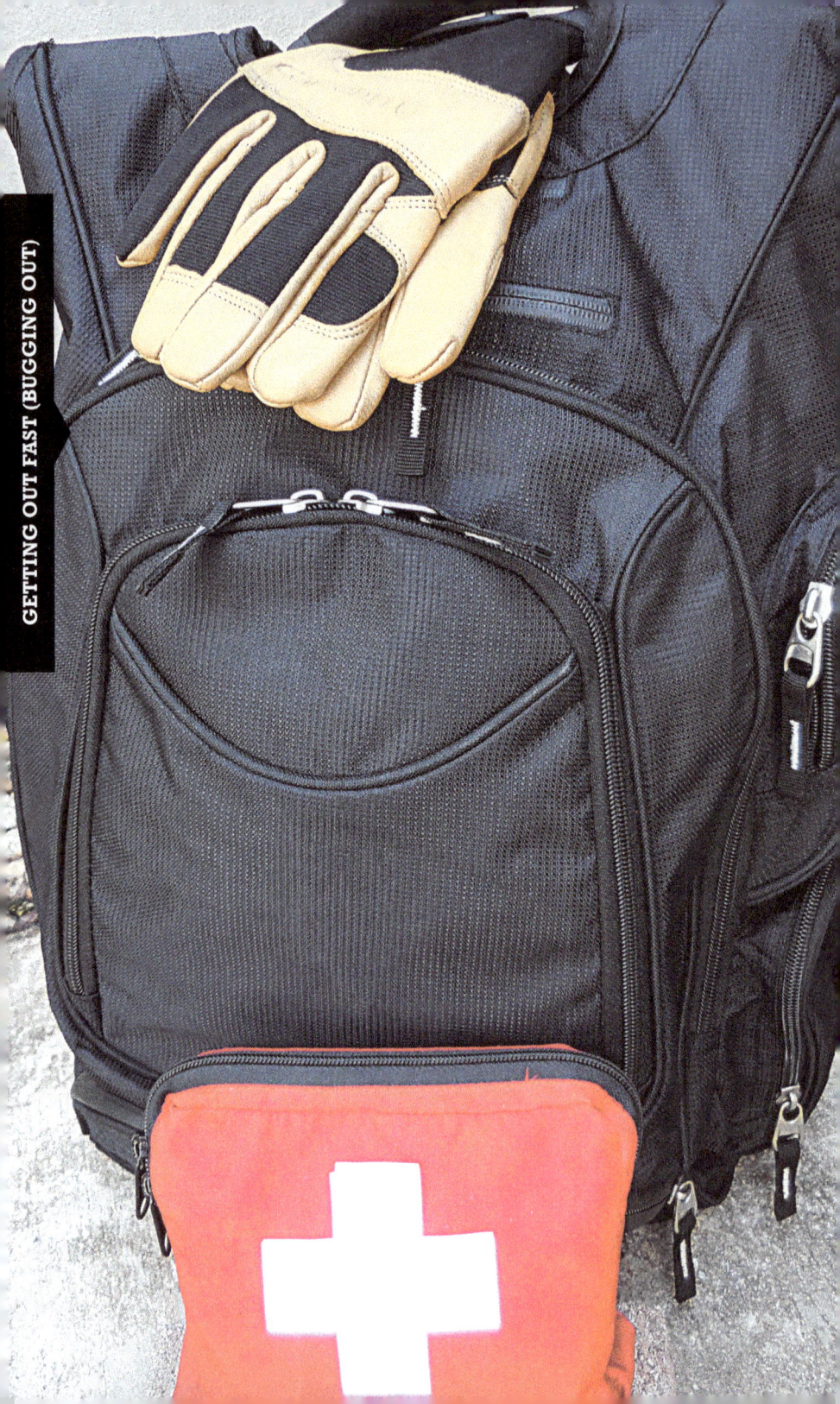

SHELTERING IN PLACE
(BUGGING IN)

WHAT TO KNOW

- Bugging in (sheltering in place) is the opposite of bugging out. It's staying put and keeping a very low profile.

- The goal of bugging in is to afford you and your group a well-stocked, secure location until it is once again safe to go outside and/or travel.

- If you are forced to bug in, chances are that the situation outside your doors will be extremely dangerous.

- In most bugging in situations, you will probably not have access to grocery stores, supermarkets, gas stations, electricity, water, or other utilities.

- A successful bug-in plan must effectively address basic survival needs—you'll need plenty of supplies. If you're not well prepared, bugging in will not be an option for you.

Quick Prep Tip

Using lights at night when the power is off will announce your presence to all around you. Do whatever you need to do during the day. At night, just lay low and remain quiet.

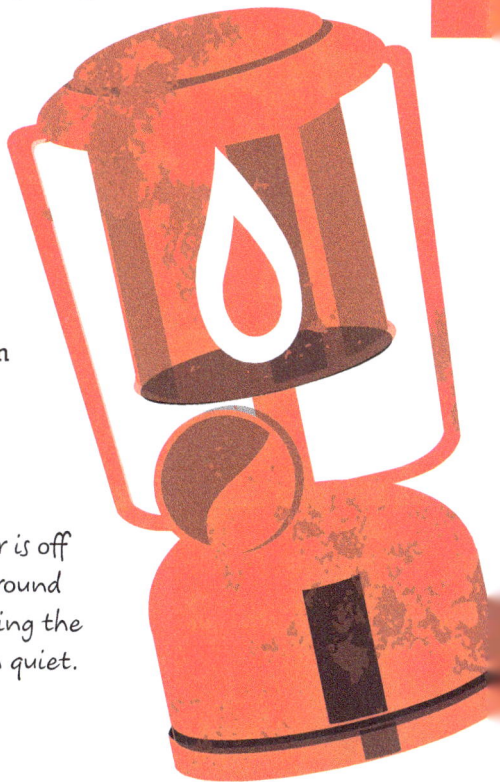

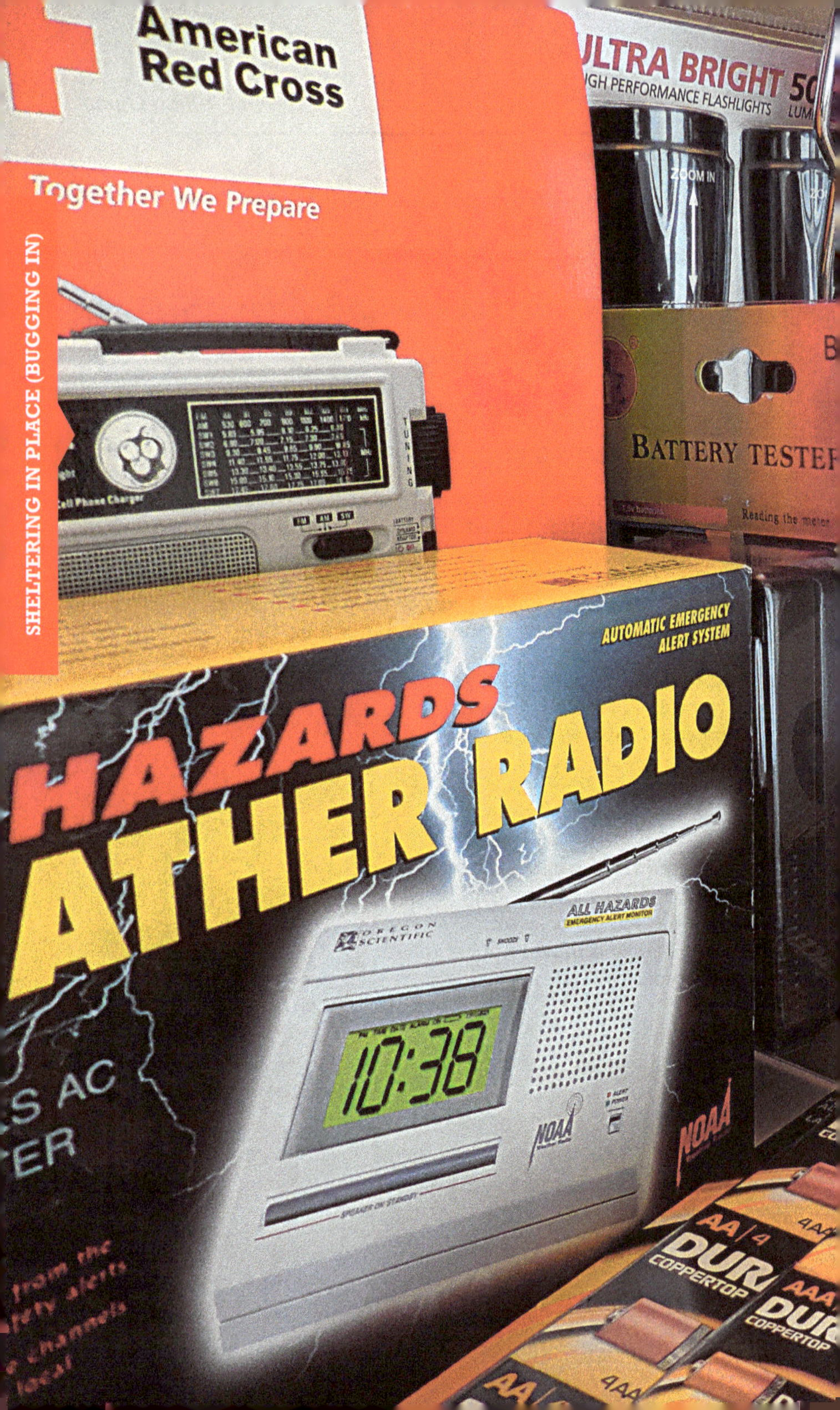
American
Red Cross
Together We Prepare
ULTRA BRIGHT
ZOOM IN
AUTOMATIC EMERGENCY
ALERT SYSTEM
HAZARDS
ATHER RADIO
ALL HAZARDS
10:38
NOAA
COPPERTOP

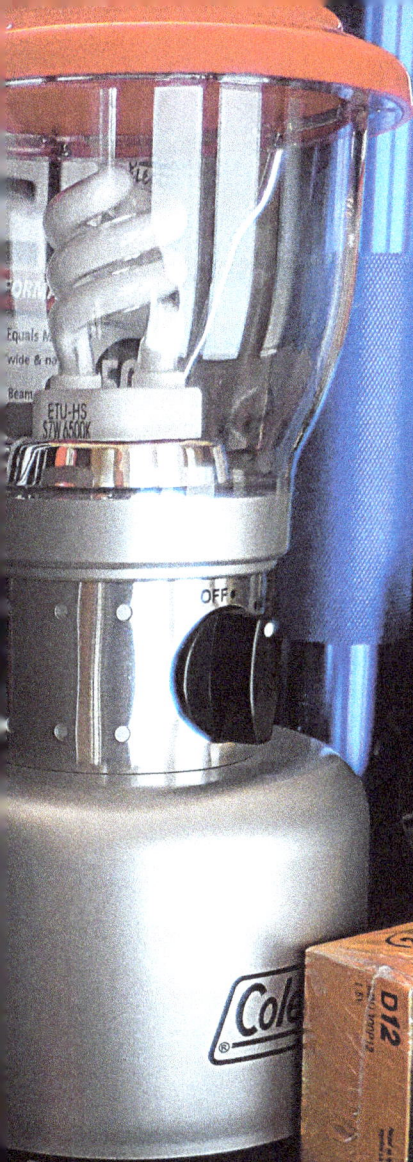

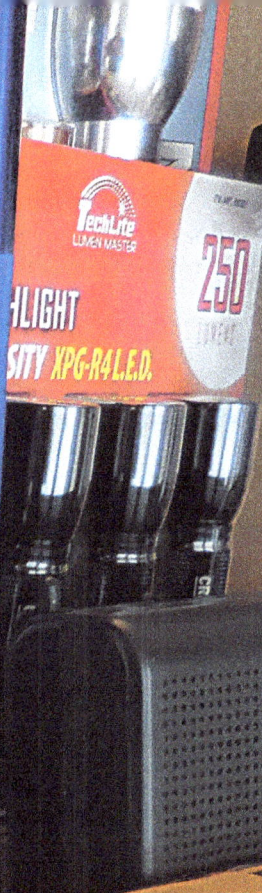

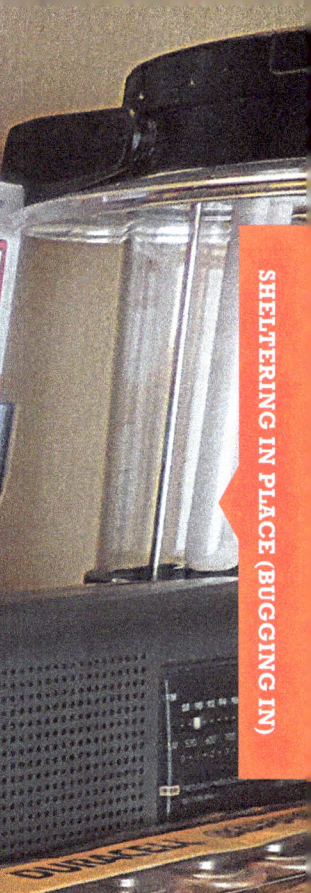

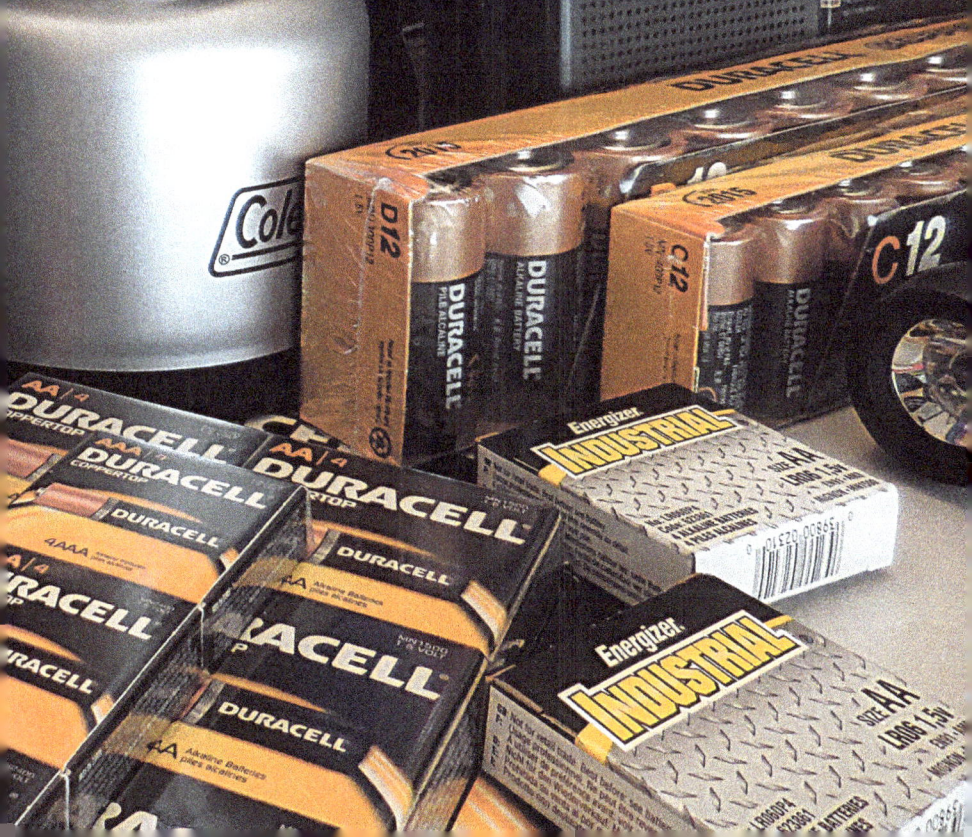

- Absent extraordinary circumstances, your home will usually be the safest place for you and your family before, during, and after a disaster.

- During a disaster, there will be plenty of desperate, hungry, thirsty people, as well as many others who will quickly take advantage of the chaotic situation to prey on the vulnerable.

- Self-defense and security play a major role in any bugging-in scenario.

WHAT TO DO

- Formulate a bugging-in plan that will allow you to take care of all your needs without leaving your location, exposing yourself, or your position. Don't neglect any special needs you or your group may have.

- Don't worry about or plan for specific threats. Plan and prepare by addressing the survival basics— food, water, first aid, security, self-defense, sanitation, and hygiene.

Quick Prep Tip

Don't cook during a bugging-in situation. The smell of food cooking can carry long distances and will broadcast to the world that you have supplies.

- Discuss your plan with all members of your group, and make sure everyone understands their role and responsibilities.

- Have a back-up plan in case your position is compromised and you are forced to leave. (Prepare a bug-out bag for each member of your group, just in case.)

- Test your plan(s) far in advance of any disaster and make adjustments as necessary.

- Stay out of sight. Remain inside your home, and keep windows and doors locked and covered.

- Don't call attention to your location—avoid lights at night, running generators, and cooking.

- Dispose of all trash/waste as securely and discretely as possible.

- Hide in plain sight. Make your location look as inconspicuous as possible. Don't do anything to call attention to yourself.

SHELTERING IN PLACE (BUGGING IN)

Quick Prep Tip

The noise from an electrical generator will announce your presence for miles and will mark you as a target of interest. In confined areas, the exhaust from a generator can be deadly. Be extremely cautious when using any sort of internal combustion generator.

WHAT TO GET

- An assortment of calorie-dense, shelf-stable foods that require no refrigeration, no cooking, and very little, if any, preparation. Simple heat-and-eat options are best. Store 2000 calories per person, per day, for no less than 90 days (see chapter 2).

- Store a minimum three-to-four-week supply of emergency, short-term bottled or tap water in water-safe containers, more if possible. Plan for at least two gallons per person, per day, for drinking. Store extra for other uses (see chapter 3).

- Firearms, a generous supply of defensive ammunition, and proper training (see chapter 4).

- First-aid and medical supplies (see chapter 5).

- A well-stocked supply of toilet paper, paper towels, disposable plates, plastic utensils, paper cups, heavy-duty plastic garbage bags, 5-gallon plastic buckets with lids, antibacterial wipes, gels, soaps, and other personal hygiene products (see chapter 6).

- Have a BOB ready to go in case circumstances cause you to abandon your location (see chapter 7).

- Communications—Have a radio (hand crank, if possible) with extra batteries.

- Flashlights, lanterns, light sticks, weather radio, extra batteries.

- Tools—Maintain an assortment of tools, gear, and equipment.

- Electrical generator—An electrical generator can be a double-edged sword. It can be a valuable asset, but it can also be a serious liability if it calls attention to your location. Have a generator with extra fuel, parts, oil, etc., but use it only when absolutely necessary and with extreme caution.

GETTING HOME
(BUGGING BACK)

WHAT TO KNOW

- If a disaster occurs while you're away from home, you need a plan and reliable access to supplies to help you get back home safely.

- During a disaster, it's not uncommon for people to be overcome with fear and shock, or to completely fall apart physically and emotionally.

- During the initial stages of a crisis, you should not expect any immediate assistance as most first responders will probably be overwhelmed.

- If you live in a densely populated urban area, your circumstances will probably be much worse as there will be a greater number of people requiring assistance and possible rescue.

- You need a plan and supplies to help you get home as quickly as possible —you need a Get-Home Bag (GHB).

- A GHB contains the supplies for self-rescue, evacuation, and getting home.

- If you don't have a GHB in your office, business, school, or vehicle, you need to get one as soon as possible.

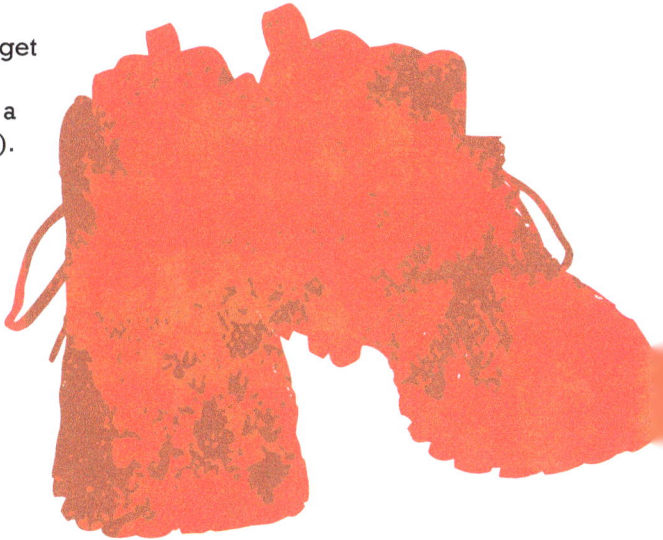

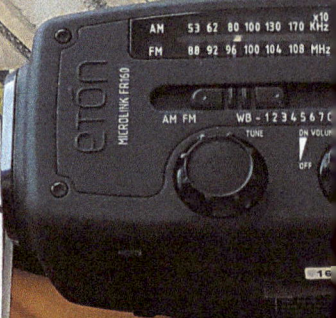
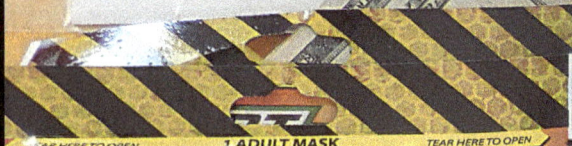
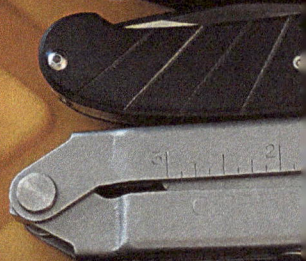
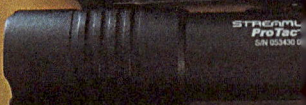
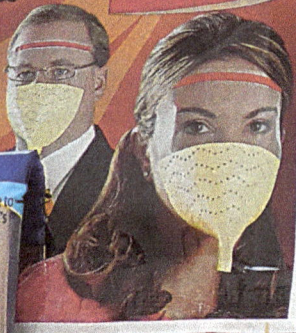
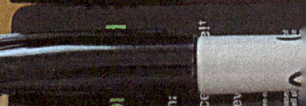

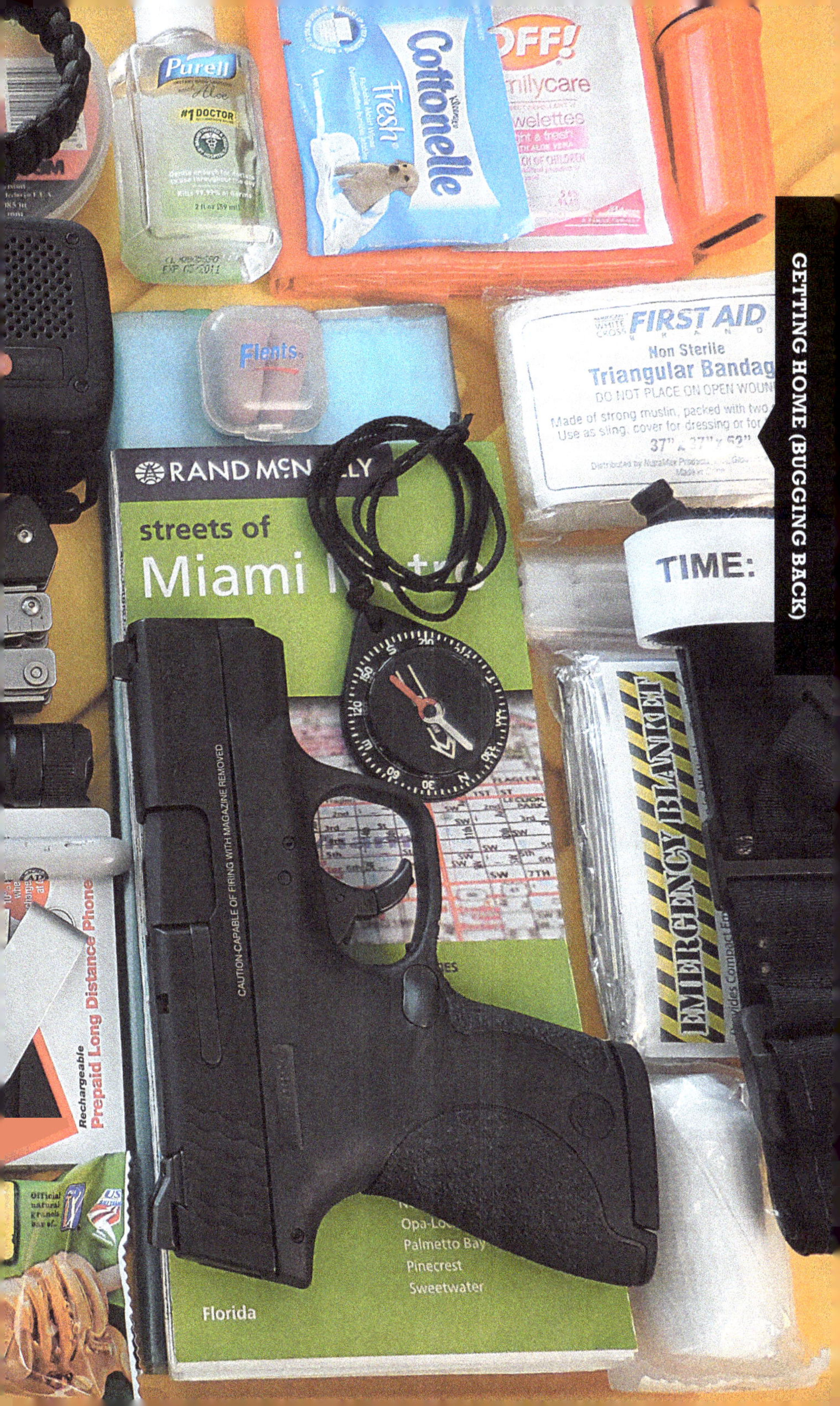
Purell
#1 DOCTOR
Cottonelle
Fresh
OFF!
milycare
FIRST AID
Non Sterile
Triangular Bandag
DO NOT PLACE ON OPEN WOUN
Made of strong muslin, packed with two
Use as sling, cover for dressing or for
Flents
RAND McN LLY
streets of
Miami
TIME:
CAUTION-CAPABLE OF FIRING WITH MAGAZINE REMOVED
EMERGENCY BLANKET
Rechargeable
Prepaid Long Distance Phone
Opa-Lo
Palmetto Bay
Pinecrest
Sweetwater
Florida

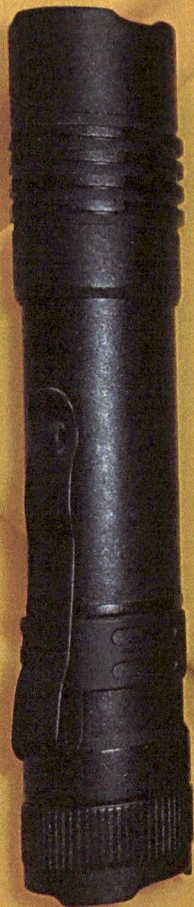

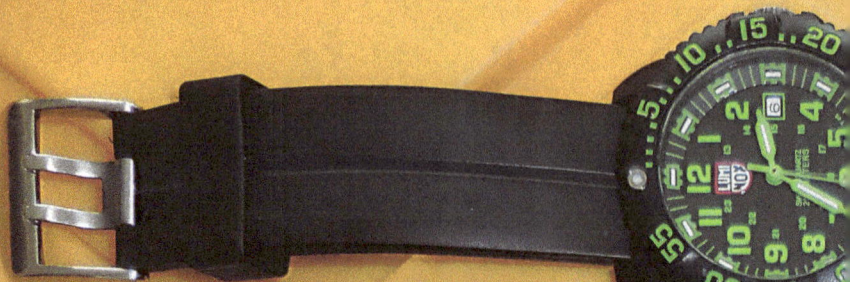

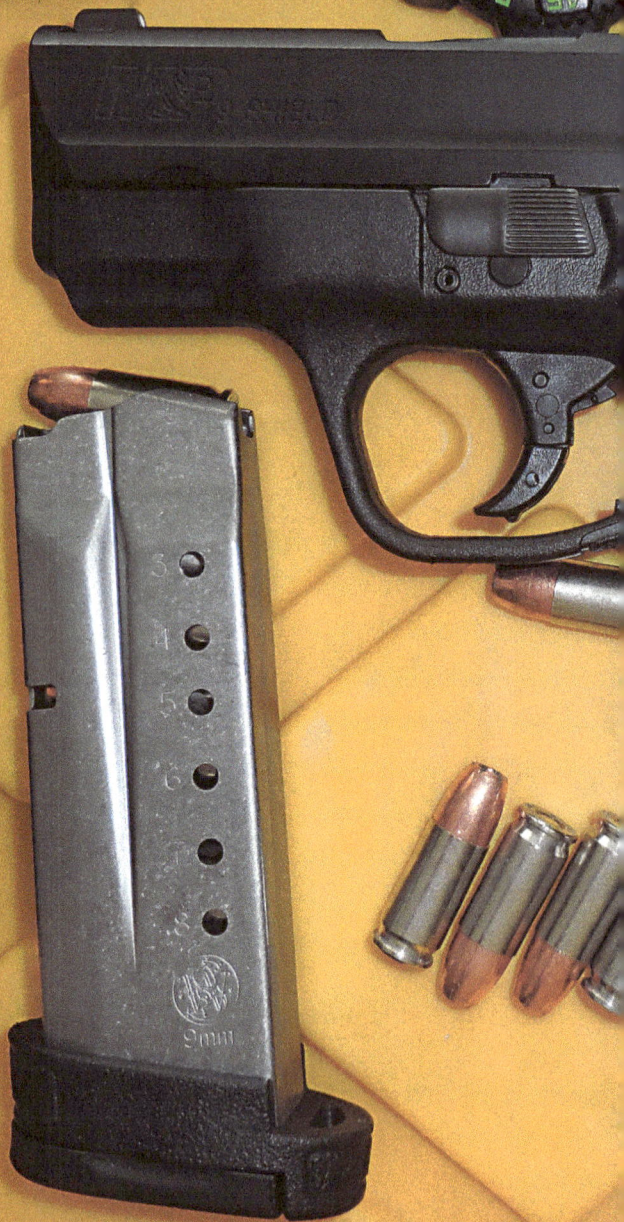

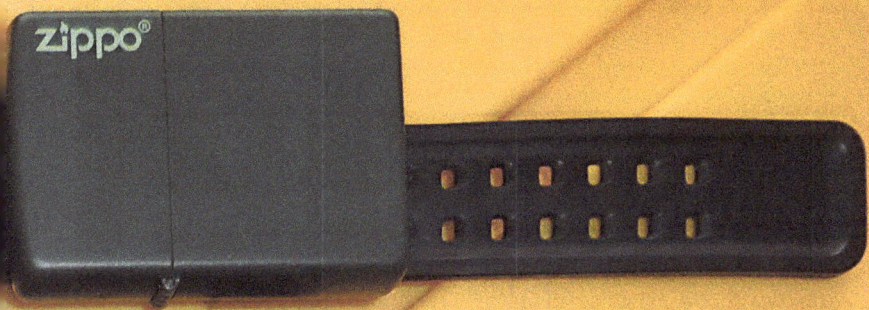
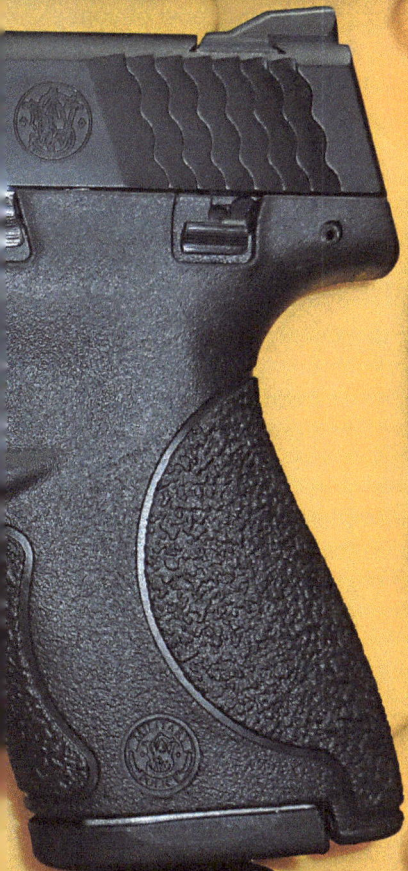
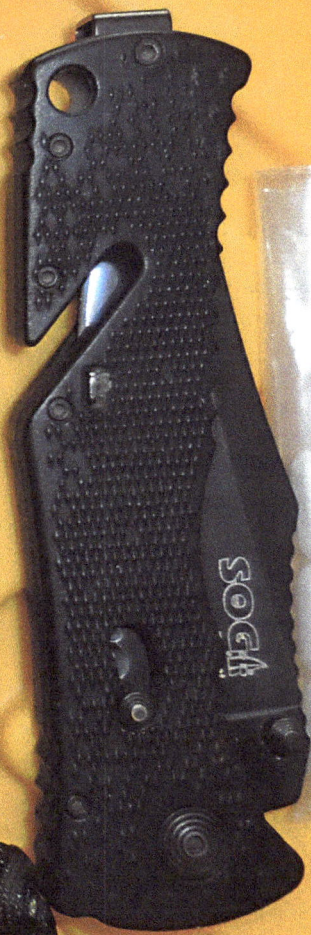
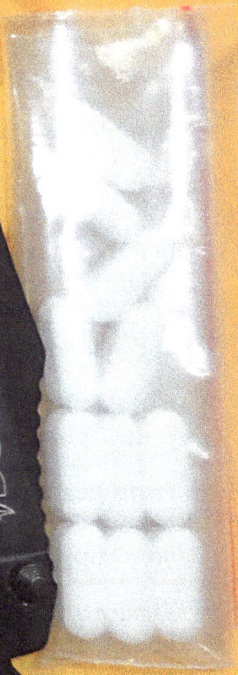
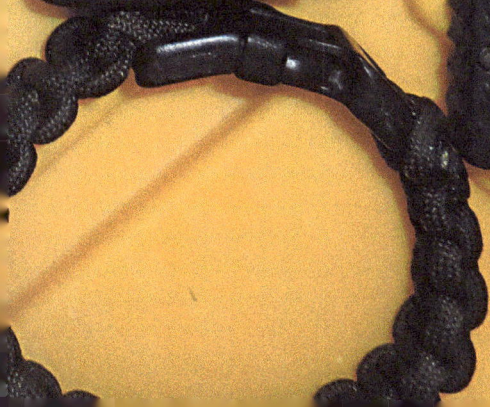

GETTING HOME (BUGGING BACK)

WHAT TO DO

- Put together a GHB with supplies that will help you get home in the aftermath of a crisis or disaster. The contents of your GHB will vary depending on your circumstances, where you spend most of your time, your medical and physical needs, and the climate where you live. Below is a list to help you get started.

- Have a get-home plan. Leave a copy of your plan and anticipated (and alternate) routes that you expect to take home. Include pre-arranged meet-up location(s) in your plan. Calculate travel distances and times.

- Find a safe and secure location to store your GHB.

- Ensure that your GHB is current and accessible at all times.

- The physical bag should be nondescript and ordinary—it should never call attention to you or to the bag itself (avoid the military or tactical look).

- Make copies of your personal documents/information (passport, driver's license, and concealed weapons permits) in case you lose your wallet/purse. Also maintain a list of all emergency contacts and phone numbers.

- Have a physical copy of all your prescription medications.

- Periodically review the contents of your GHB; rotate and update your supplies often.

- Ensure all members of your household have a GHB that is appropriate for their situation, age, and abilities.

Quick Prep Tip

The items in a GHB should not be confused with Every Day Carry (EDC) items. EDC items should always be on your person and typically include a weapon, a pocketknife, a flashlight, and a small supply of emergency medication, a phone, etc.

WHAT TO GET

- **Medium-sized book bag** (or similar style of bag) with comfortable carrying straps and easily accessible compartments. Black or a similar dark color is best to avoid attracting attention.

- **High-output LED flashlight, headlamp with extra batteries.** Also consider glow sticks.

- **First aid kit/medical supplies**—small supply of everything you may need.

- **Prescription medication** (no less than 72 hours, more if possible).

- **Potassium iodide tablets**, to protect your thyroid gland from radiation.

- **Sunscreen and bug repellent (if applicable).**

- **N95masks, goggles, gloves, earplugs, extra pair of prescription glasses.**

- **Pocket knife and/or multi-tool.**

- **Radio** (hand crank preferred) or with extra batteries.

Quick Prep Tip

Always keep the contents of your GHB current; rotate your supplies often. Test your equipment periodically to ensure it's working properly. Remember, the day you need it, you will need it desperately.

- **Bottled water, energy bars, small portable water filter.**

- **Hand wipes, antibacterial gel, travel-size roll of toilet paper.**

- **Rain gear, poncho, extra clothes, hat, and comfortable walking shoes/boots.**

- **Moleskin**—to protect feet when walking long distances.

- **Cash (small bills and some coins)**—at least $250.00.

- **Compass and map** of your expected travel area(s) with locations of interest (hospitals, police stations, fire stations, and water sources) clearly marked.

- **Duct tape, re-sealable plastic bags, 550 Paracord (50').**

- **Personal protection**—lethal or non-lethal, depending on your circumstances.

- **Pre-paid calling card** (in case your cell phone is lost/damaged, or if service is down).

- **List of contact information,** phone numbers, addresses, etc.

- **Water-resistant bag** to store copies of your important documents and papers.

The only purpose of a GHB is to help you get home. The list above is just a starting point, and you'll need to adjust your GHB to your particular needs and circumstances.

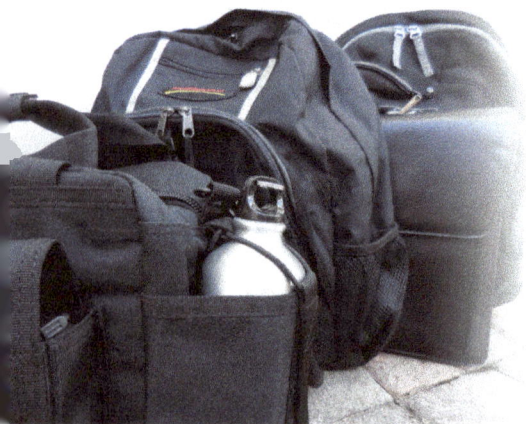

EMERGENCY VEHICLE KIT

WHAT TO KNOW

- Drivers need to plan and prepare for roadside emergencies.

- A prepared driver will keep a fully stocked Emergency Vehicle Kit (EVK) in their vehicle at all times.

- The contents of your EVK will depend on your circumstances, where you live, and the type of roads you normally drive on.

- The most important thing, however, is to have a kit with supplies, gear, and equipment to help you survive a roadside emergency.

WHAT TO DO

- Start with a basic kit and expand it as your needs change.

- Having tools and supplies is important, but you should also focus on learning the skills that will help you during a roadside emergency.

- Keep your vehicle in good repair and perform tune-ups, oil changes, and routine maintenance as required.

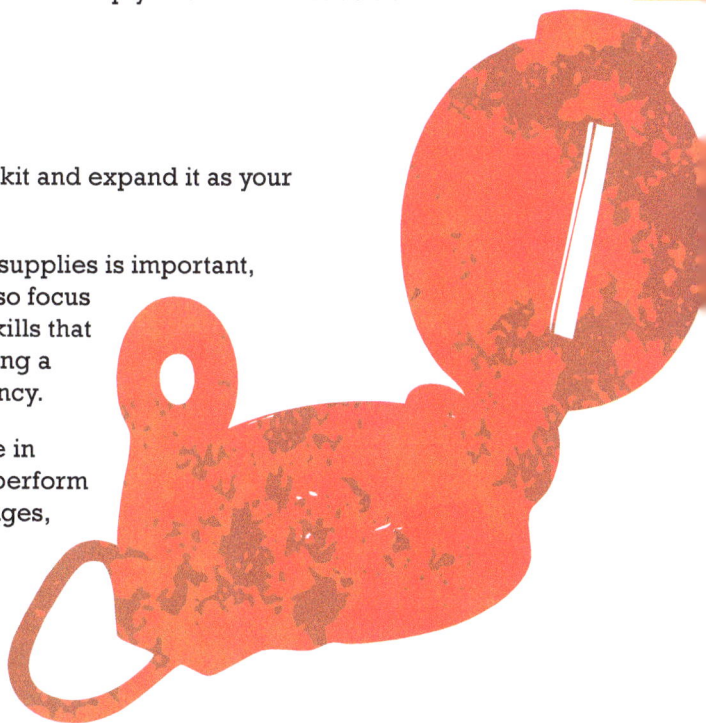

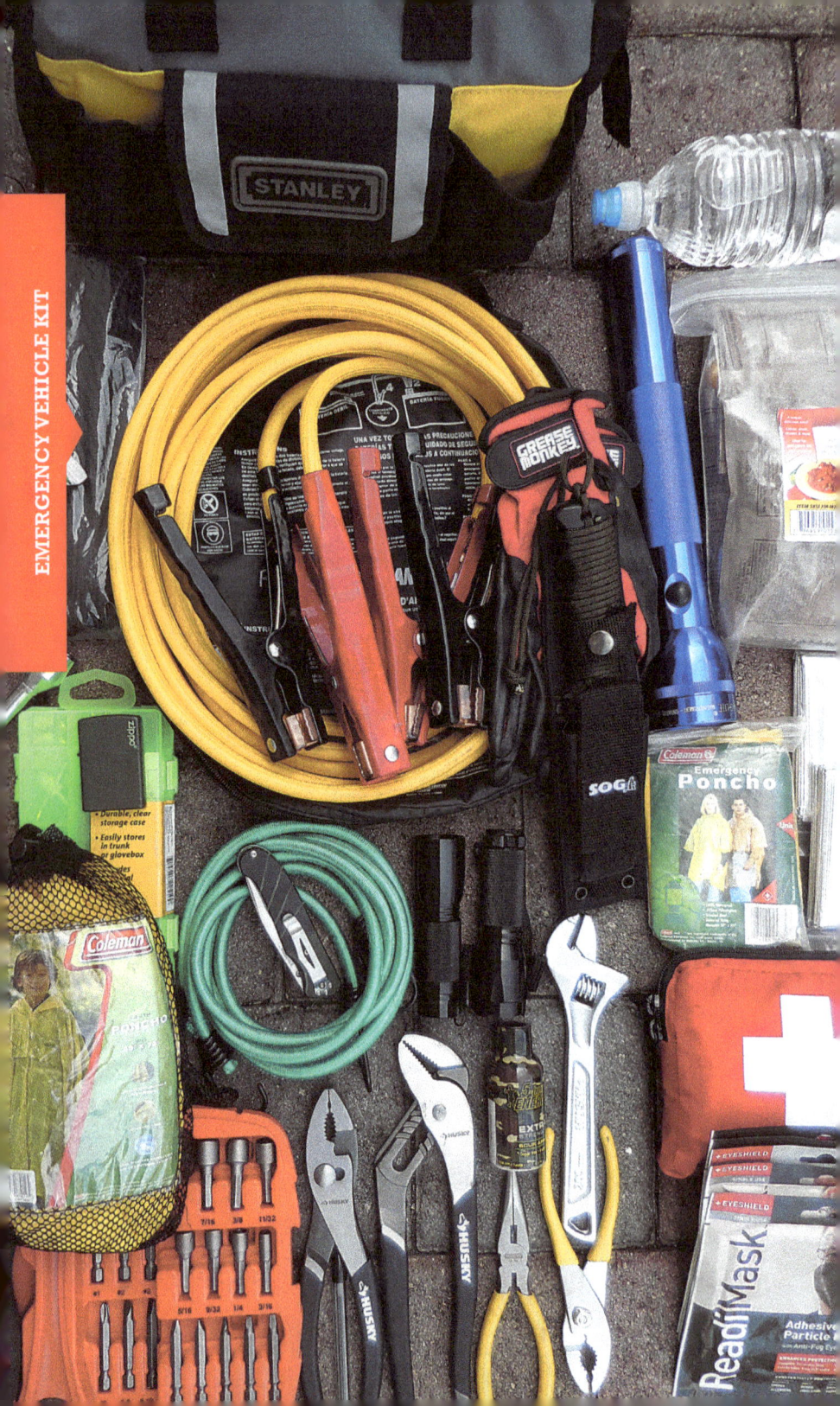

EMERGENCY VEHICLE KIT

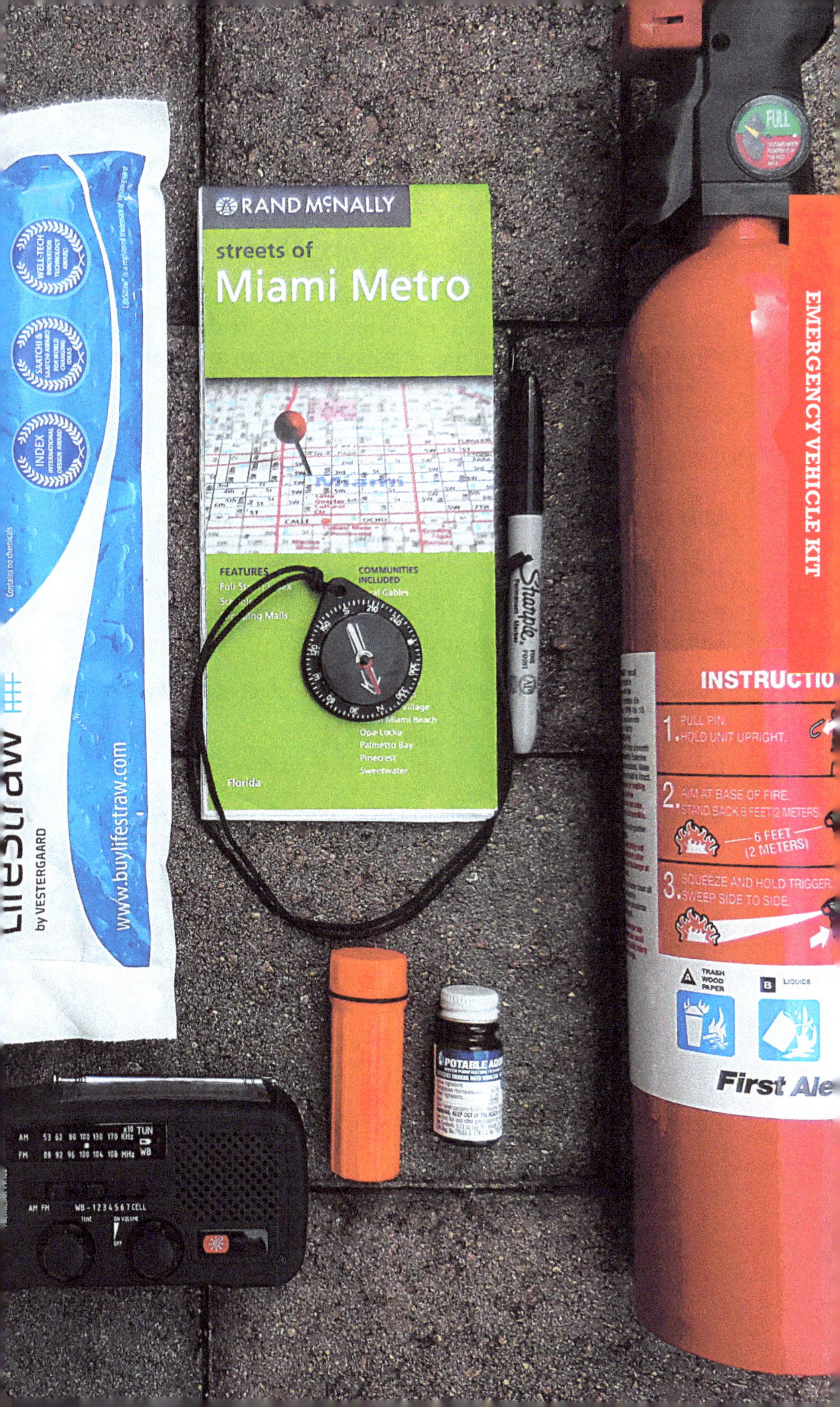

- Learn to read road maps and navigate using a compass.

- Stay in good physical health. All survival situations will be more manageable if you're in good health.

- Always leave a copy of your plans and anticipated travel routes with a friend, relative, or neighbor. If you don't return as scheduled, they will at least know where to start looking for you.

WHAT TO GET

- **LED flashlight/lantern** with a supply of extra batteries.

- **Light sticks**—Large light sticks.

- **Road flares**—Quality road flares stored in a waterproof container or electronic LED-type road flares.

- **Basic hand tools**—Screwdrivers, pliers, wrenches, socket set, etc.

- **Air compressor, supplies, and tools to fix a flat tire.**

- **Battery jumper cables**—Quality cables (8-12 feet long)

Quick Prep Tip

Review the contents of your EVK on a regular basis. Update and rotate supplies as needed.

- **Gloves and eye protection**—Impact resistant eye protection and heavy-duty gloves.

- **First-aid kit**—Maintain quality supplies and know how to use them.

- **Prescriptions**—Keep a copy of prescriptions and at least a three-day supply of any medicine you take.

- **Folding knife and quality multi-tool.**

- **Folding shovel**, emergency digging tool.

- **Electrical/duct tape, tie wraps.**

- **Space blankets**—Multi-purpose blankets are inexpensive and easy to use.

- **Map of your travel area, compass, note pad, and pens.**

- **Reading glasses**—Back-up to your primary pair.

- **Water and non-perishable emergency food**—Store food and water for two people for a minimum of three days. Open-and-eat, calorie-dense food options are best.

- **Five-gallon gas can (empty) with a siphon.**

EMERGENCY VEHICLE KIT

Quick Prep Tip

Don't wait until you have a flat tire to find out that your jack is missing pieces or that your spare tire is damaged.

EMERGENCY VEHICLE KIT

- **Cash**—Small bills and some coins.

- **Duct and electrical tape, 550 Paracord (at least 100 feet).**

- **Fire extinguisher**—Class B (for liquids and gases) and Class C (for energized electrical equipment).

- **Extra set of clothing, hat, jacket, and gloves**—Climate-specific and adjusted seasonally.

- **Extra pair of comfortable walking shoes**—Climate-specific, comfortable, and durable walking or hiking shoes/boots.

- **Towels**—Multiple sizes.

- **Self-defense tools**—Protection against threats, human or otherwise.

- **Whistle, fire starter, and signal mirror**—Especially if you frequent rural areas.

- **Contact information**—Hard copy of important and emergency contact numbers.

- **Calling card**—For use on a pay phone or a landline, especially when traveling out of your area code.

Quick Prep Tip

Maintain your vehicle in good repair. Perform routine maintenance to avoid bigger problems later on.

LEGAL AND FINANCIAL PREPARATIONS

WHAT TO KNOW

- Every crisis, no matter how severe, has always been followed by a rebuilding and reconstruction phase.

- There will be insurance claims to be filed, repairs to be made, banks, creditors, utilities, and insurance companies to call. There will be lots of time-consuming bureaucracy to deal with.

- While many legal and financial documents are stored and recorded electronically by third-party institutions, getting access to copies after a disaster may not be possible.

- Recovery and reconstruction is tremendously difficult (if not impossible), without access to your legal, financial, and insurance information and documents.

- Dealing with the aftermath of a disaster will be easier if you take the time to identify, organize, copy, and secure your personal and business documents, records, and information.

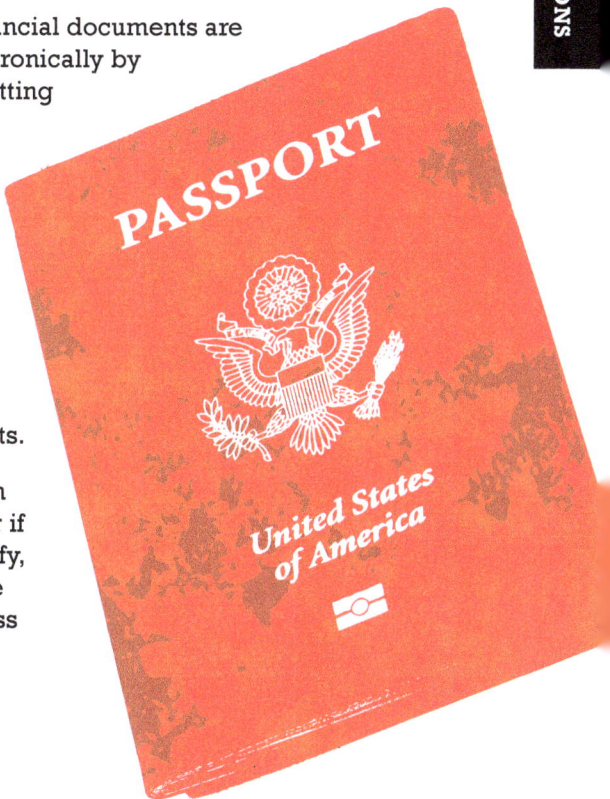

INCORPORATED UNDER THE
THE STATE OF FLORIDA

SATISFACTION OF

PASSPOR

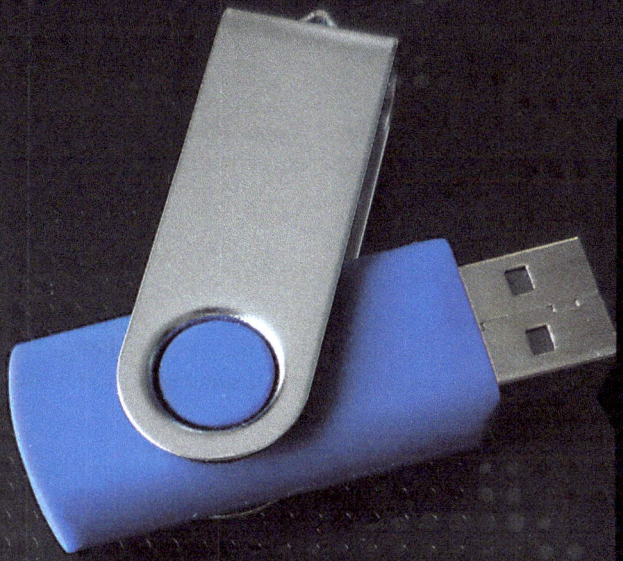

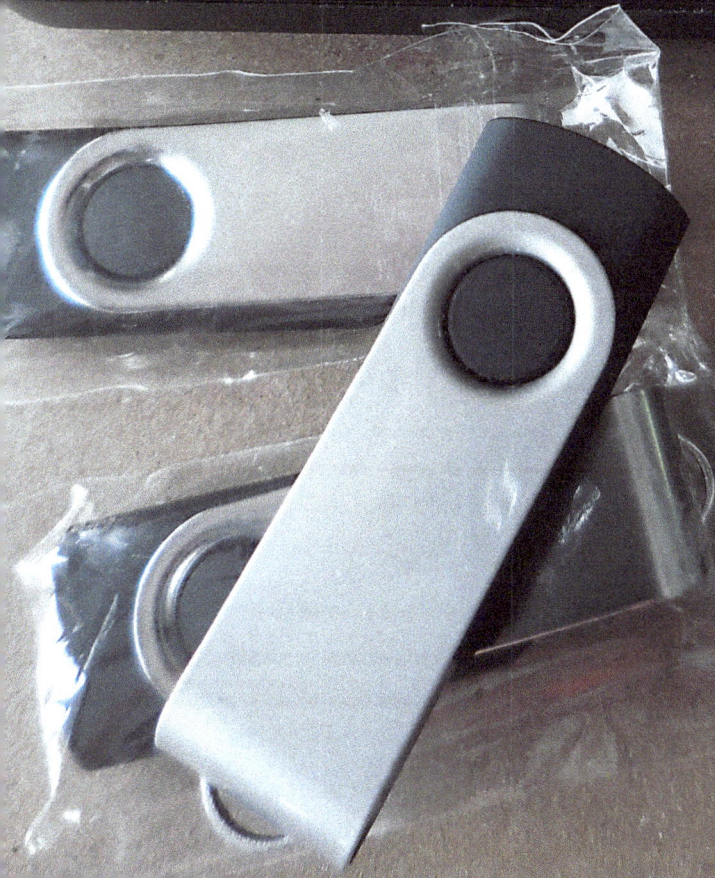

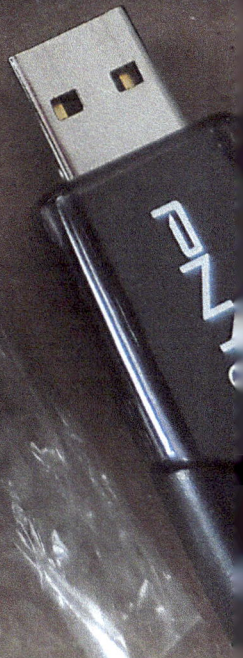

- Trying to replace important records and documents after a disaster will be extremely difficult and in some instances, next to impossible.

WHAT TO DO

- Focus on securing the legal and financial components that will form the basis of your reconstruction and rebuilding efforts in the aftermath of a crisis.

- Identify, secure, and copy all your legal, financial, and insurance documents, records, files, and information.

- Prioritize your documents and information into three separate categories as follows: crucial, important, and nice-to-have. Focus your efforts accordingly.

- Use password-protected storage devices and encryption software to help protect your information, documents, and images.

Quick Prep Tip

Use a password that includes a combination of no less than fifteen (15) upper and lower case letters, numbers, and symbols. Avoid using names, birthdays, telephone numbers, addresses, or other commonly known information.

- Secure all personal information and documents against damage, destruction, and theft. Limit access to only a small and trusted group of individuals.

- Store originals in fireproof, waterproof containers.

- Secure copies (paper/digital) in redundant locations.

- Maintain portable, secure storage devices and hardcopies that will allow quick and easy access to your records for bugging out or other such emergencies.

- Maintain an alternate off-site storage location in the event that your primary location is somehow compromised or unavailable to you.

- Copy and scan all documents and papers for safekeeping.

- Record and secure all key information and documents.

- Consider securing a bank safe-deposit box to serve as off-premise storage for original documents. A safe-deposit box will probably not be accessible during a crisis, but your documents will be secure, and you can make back-up copies to keep at home.

Quick Prep Tip

A portable (grab-and-go)
hard drive is an effective
way to back up and store
your most important
files. Protect your data
with a password.

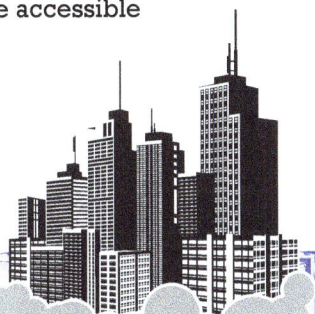

LEGAL AND FINANCIAL PREPARATIONS

WHAT TO GET

- **Portable disc drive and flash drives/thumb drives.**

- **Waterproof document case.**

- **Lockable, fire/water-resistant safe or file cabinet.**

- **Mylar bags.** One-gallon size works well to store and provide a waterproof seal for standard size (8.5 X 11) documents.

Quick Prep Tip

Flash drives are effective, inexpensive, and hold lots of data.

About The Author

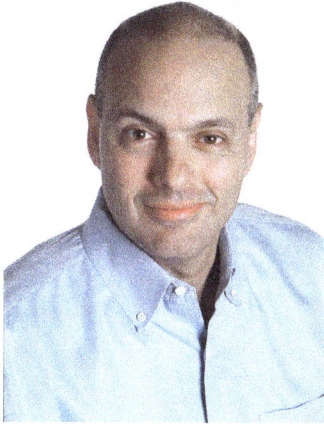

Richard Duarte is the author of *Surviving Doomsday: A Guide for Surviving an Urban Disaster.* He's a practicing attorney and an avid firearms enthusiast. Richard lectures and consults in the areas of urban survival planning and preparation, and is a contributing writer for a number of firearms and preparedness publications. As a father, grandfather, husband, and responsible member of society, he refuses to delegate responsibility for his family's welfare and safety, and passionately promotes self-reliance and preparedness. When he's not writing, speaking, teaching, or thinking about urban preparedness, he's busy running his law office in Miami, Florida.

For the latest news and updates, you can connect with Richard on Facebook, Twitter, and his blog.

www.survivingdoomsdaythebook.com

www.facebook.com/survivingdoomsdaythebook

www.twitter.com/SurvivingDoomsd

"There are no guarantees in life, but after any major disaster, two separate and distinct groups will emerge—the Prepared and the Unprepared. It's up to you which group you'll belong to. As far as I'm concerned, the ultimate measure of this book's success will be how many people it can help guide into the 'prepared' group."

– Richard Duarte

"Stay Safe and Be Prepared!"

SHARE YOUR EXPERIENCE

Please take a moment to post a review on Amazon.com.

Others will appreciate your thoughts and insights.